Last Minute Intercollegiate MRCS Applied Basic Science Questions

Samena Chaudhry MRCS (Eng)

SHO Trauma and Orthopaedics
Stafford District General Hospital
Stafford

Sandipan Pati MBBS

SHO Neurosurgery
Department of Neuroscience/Neurology
University Hospital of North Staffordshire
Stoke on Trent

Tahseen Chaudhry BMedSc (physiology) MBChB

SHO Trauma and Orthopaedics
Department of Trauma and Orthopaedics
Royal Shrewsbury Hospital
Shrewsbury

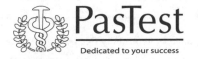

PasTest

Dedicated to your success

© 2006 PASTEST LTD
Egerton Court
Parkgate Estate
Knutsford
Cheshire
WA16 8DX

Telephone: 01565 752000

First Published 2006

ISBN: 1 904627 64 1
ISBN: 978 1904627 647

A catalogue record for this book is available from the British Library.

The information contained within this book was obtained by the author from reliable sources. However, while every effort has been made to ensure its accuracy, no responsibility for loss, damage or injury occasioned to any person acting or refraining from action as a result of information contained herein can be accepted by the publishers or authors.

PasTest Revision Books and Intensive Courses

PasTest has been established in the field of postgraduate medical education since 1972, providing revision books and intensive study courses for doctors preparing for their professional examinations.

Books and courses are available for the following specialties:

MRCGP, MRCP Parts 1 and 2, MRCPCH Parts 1 and 2, MRCPsych, MRCS, MRCOG Parts 1 and 2, DRCOG, DCH, FRCA, PLAB Parts 1 and 2.

For further details contact:

PasTest, Freepost, Knutsford, Cheshire WA16 7BR

Tel: 01565 752000   Fax: 01565 650264
www.pastest.co.uk   enquiries@pastest.co.uk

Text typeset and designed by Type Study, Scarborough, North Yorkshire

Printed and bound in the UK by Alden Group Limited, Oxfordshire

CONTENTS

CONTRIBUTORS

JB Elder

Professor in General Surgery
University of Keele, Stoke on Trent

N Maffulli

Professor of Trauma and Orthopaedics
University of Keele, Stoke on Trent

Mrs C Hall

Consultant in General Surgery
University Hospital North Staffordshire

Mr AS Jaipersad

Specialist Registrar in General Surgery
University Hospital North Staffordshire

Balasubramanian Chandramanian

Specialist Registrar in Neurosurgery
University Hospital North Staffordshire

Quang Ngyugen

Senior House Officer in ENT
University Hospital North Staffordshire

Yew Wei Tan

Senior House Officer in Accident and Emergency
University Hospital North Staffordshire

Veenoo Agarwal

Senior House Officer in General Surgery
University Hospital North Staffordshire

FOREWORD

This book is especially written for MRCS candidates taking their Applied Basic Science paper at the Intercollegiate level. The editors and contributors have been either recent successful candidates themselves or are examiners. While the questions do cover the three classical areas of anatomy, physiology and pathology, the truly modern and refreshing additions in this book are the helpful explanations accompanying many of the questions.

It is, therefore, a book which aims to educate the reader by filling in gaps in his or her knowledge and is far more than just a collection of relevant questions. The book will serve many and help them to pass their examinations with a clearer understanding of the basic science so necessary for the modern young surgeon. I congratulate the editors and PasTest publishers on producing this very helpful book for candidates who are very often working in full time jobs as well as preparing for this examination. Clearing the necessary and mandatory hurdle in their pursuit of a surgical career will undoubtedly be easier for those using this book. It has been a privilege and a pleasure for me to be involved in the enterprise and I wholeheartedly commend it to all those intending to sit the MRCS examination.

JB Elder, Emeritus Professor of Surgery, Keele University Medical School
May 2006

ABBREVIATIONS

AAA	aortic artery aneurysm
ABI	ankle–brachial index
ACE	angiotensin-converting enzyme
ACL	anterior cruciate ligament
ACTH	adrenocorticotrophic hormone
ADH	antidiuretic hormone
AFP	α-fetoprotein
ALP	alkaline phosphatase
ARDS	acute respiratory distress syndrome
AV	atrioventricular
BCC	basal cell carcinoma
CCK	cholecystokinin
CEA	carcinoembryonic antigen
CES	cauda equina syndrome
CN	cranial nerve
CRP	C-reactive protein
CPP	cerebral perfusion pressure
CST	cavernous sinus thrombosis
CSF	cerebrospinal fluid
CT	computed tomography
CTZ	chemoreceptor trigger zone
CT	computed tomography
CVP	central venous pressure
DAT	direct anti-globulin test
DRE	digital rectal examination
2,3-DPG	2,3-diphosphoglycerate
DVT	deep venous thrombosis
EBV	Epstein–Barr virus
ECA	external cartoid artery
ESR	erythrocyte sedimentation rate
ECF	extracellular fluid
EJV	external jugular vein
FDP	flexor digitorum profundus
FDS	flexor digitorum superficialis
FEV_1	forced expiratory volume in 1 s
FNA	fine-needle aspiration
FRC	functional residual capacity
FSH	follicle-stimulating hormone
GABA	γ-aminobutyric acid
GCS	Glasgow Coma Score
GFR	glomerular filtration rate
GORD	gastro-oesophageal reflux disease
HAV	hepatitis A virus
HBV	hepatitis B virus
HCV	hepatitis C virus
β-hCG	β-human chorionic gonadotrophin
HDL	high-density lipoprotein

HIV	human immunodeficiency virus
HPGRT	hypoxanthine–guanine–phosphoribosyltransferase
HPV	human papillomavirus
HZV	herpes zoster virus
ICA	internal carotid artery
ICP	intracerebral pressure or intracranial pressure
ITU	intensive therapy unit
IVC	inferior vena cava
JVP	jugular venous pressure
LCA	lateral cricoarytenoid
LCL	lateral collateral ligament
LDL	low-density lipoprotein
LH	luteinising hormone
LMW	low-molecular-weight
LVEDV	left ventricular end-diastolic volume
LVF	left ventricular failure
MAP	mean arterial pressure
MCL	medial cruciate ligament
MCH	mean cell haemoglobin
MCV	mean cell volume
MMA	middle meningeal artery
MRI	magnetic resonance imaging
MRSA	methicillin-resistant *Staphylococcus aureus*
NSAIDs	non-steroidal anti-inflammatory drugs
PAH	*p*-aminohippuric acid
PCA	posterior cricoarytenoid or patient-controlled analgesia
PCL	posterior cruciate ligament
P_{CO_2}	partial pressure of carbon dioxide
PE	pulmonary embolism
PEEP	positive end-expiratory pressure
P_{O_2}	partial pressure of oxygen
PSA	prostate-specific antigen
RBCs	red blood cells
REM	rapid eye movement
RLN	recurrent laryngeal nerve
RPF	renal plasma flow
RV	residual volume
SCC	squamous cell carcinoma
SCM	sternocleidomastoid
SIRS	systemic inflammatory response syndrome
SLN	superior laryngeal nerve
SVC	superior vena cava
T_3	triiodothyronine
T_4	thyroxine
TENS	transcutaneous electrical nerve stimulation
TGF	transforming growth factor
TLC	total lung capacity
TM	tympanic membrane
TMJ	temporomandibular joint
TPN	total parenteral nutrition
TPO	thyroid peroxidase
TRH	thyroid-releasing hormone
TSH	thyroid-stimulating hormone
VC	vital capacity

vCJD	variant Creutzfeldt–Jakob disease
VF	ventricular fibrillation
VIP	vasoactive poplypeptide
VLDL	very-low-density lipoprotein
VT	ventricular tachycardia

1. ANATOMY

Multiple true/false questions

1.1 **The phrenic nerve(s):**

- [ ] **A** Are formed from anterior primary rami of spinal nerves C3, C4, C5 and C6.
- [ ] **B** Are the sole motor supply to the diaphragm.
- [ ] **C** Are accompanied by the pericardicophrenic vessels.
- [ ] **D** On the right, descends on the right of the inferior vena cava (IVC) to the diaphragm where it passes through close to the caval opening.
- [ ] **E** On the right, pierces the diaphragm anterior to the central tendon.

1.2 **With regard to the scalene muscles:**

- [ ] **A** The anterior scalene muscle descends from the transverse processes of C3.
- [ ] **B** The middle scalene muscle inserts on the under-surface of the first rib.
- [ ] **C** The posterior scalene muscle passes from the transverse process of C5 through C7 to the lateral surface of the second rib.
- [ ] **D** The subclavian arteries are separated from the veins by the anterior scalene muscle.
- [ ] **E** C3, C4 and C5 spinal nerves emerge between the middle and posterior scalene muscles.

1.1　Answer: B, C, D

The phrenic nerve on both sides originates from C3, C4 and C5. It descends on the anterio-surface of scalenus anterior before crossing the subclavian artery and entering the thorax. The right phrenic nerve pierces the diaphragm in its tendinous portion just slightly lateral to the IVC foramen. The left passes via the left leaf of the diaphragm.

1.2　Answer: A, C, D

The anterior scalene muscle descends inferolaterally from the transverse processes of C3–C6 to the scalene tubercle on the first rib. The middle scalene muscle descends inferolaterally from the transverse processes of C2–C7 to the upper surface of the first rib. The posterior scalene muscle passes from the transverse process of C5–C7 to the lateral surface of the second rib. The subclavian arteries are separated from the veins by the anterior scalene muscle.

1.3 **The subclavian artery:**

☐ **A** Has a first part that is medial to the anterior scalene muscle.

☐ **B** Has a second part that lies anterior to the anterior scalene muscle.

☐ **C** Has a costocervical trunk arising from its anterior aspect.

☐ **D** Has a suprascapular artery that is a branch of the thyrocervical trunk.

☐ **E** Has a transverse cervical artery that gives branches to trapezius.

1.3   Answer: A, D, E

The *first part of the subclavian artery* has three branches.

First branch: the vertebral artery has two parts – the cervical and suboccipital. Its cervical part ascends just medial to the muscles and passes deeply at its apex, to course through the foramina of the transverse processes of C1–C6. The suboccipital part courses in a groove on the posterior arch of the atlas before it enters the cranial cavity through the foramen magnum.

Second branch: the internal thoracic artery arises from the anteroinferior aspect of the subclavian artery and passes inferomedially into the thorax. The cervical part of this artery has no branches.

Third branch: the thyrocervical trunk arises from the anterosuperior aspect of the first part of the subclavian artery, just medial to the anterior scalene muscle, and divides into the:

(1) inferior thyroid artery
(2) suprascapular artery
(3) transverse cervical artery.

It gives off branches to muscles in the posterior cervical triangle, trapezius and medial scapular muscles.

The *second part of the subclavian artery* is posterior to the anterior scalene muscle and has only one branch: the costocervical trunk, which arises from the posterior aspect of the subclavian artery. It passes posterosuperiorly and divides into the superior intercostal artery and the deep cervical arteries. It supplies the posterior deep cervical muscles.

The *third part of the subclavian artery* is lateral to the anterior scalene muscle and only has one branch: the dorsal scapular artery.

1.4 Structures passing through the foramen magnum include:

- [ ] A The anterior spinal artery.
- [ ] B The dura.
- [ ] C The vagus nerve.
- [ ] D The spinal accessory nerve.
- [ ] E The vertebral artery.

1.5 Nerves that pass in the lateral wall of the cavernous sinus include:

- [ ] A The ophthalmic division of the trigeminal nerve.
- [ ] B The sixth cranial nerve.
- [ ] C The posterior ethmoidal nerve.
- [ ] D The optic nerve.
- [ ] F The third cranial nerve.

1.6 Damage to cranial nerve XII in the hypoglossal canal causes:

- [ ] A Atrophy of the same side of the tongue.
- [ ] B Deviation of the tongue to the same side on protrusion.
- [ ] C Impaired closure of the oropharyngeal isthmus.
- [ ] D Impaired depression of the hyoid bone.
- [ ] E Paralysis of the extrinsic, but not the intrinsic, muscles of the same side of the tongue.

1.7 The postsynaptic, sympathetic and parasympathetic fibres from the pterygopalatine (sphenopalatine) ganglion innervate:

- [ ] A The lacrimal gland.
- [ ] B The iris.
- [ ] C The parotid gland.
- [ ] D The submandibular gland.
- [ ] E The glands in the mucosa of the maxillary air sinus.

1.4 **Answer: A, B, D, E**

The *vagus nerve* runs through the jugular foramen.

1.5 **Answer: none of them**

The *cavernous sinus* lies between the cranial and meningeal layers of the dura mater in relation to the body of the sphenoid bone. The cranial nerves III, IV and V in its lateral wall. Running within it are the internal carotid artery and cranial nerve VI.

1.6 **Answer: A, B**

If there is damage to the *hypoglossal nerve*, there is deviation towards the side of injury. In addition, there is flaccid paralysis and atrophy of the tongue muscles, as well as fasciculation.

If damage occurs to the corticobulbar tract, the tongue deviates to the opposite side of the lesion.

1.7 **Answer: A, E**

The postsynaptic, parasympathetic and sympathetic fibres pass to the lacrimal gland and the glands of the nasal cavity, palate and upper pharynx.

1.8 The pterygopalatine ganglion provides motor supply to the:

☐ **A** Lacrimal gland.

☐ **B** Nasal mucosa.

☐ **C** Palatine glands.

☐ **D** Mucosa of nasal pharynx posterior to the auditory tube.

☐ **E** Parotid gland.

1.9 Branches of the maxillary artery include:

☐ **A** The inferior alveolar artery.

☐ **B** The posterior superior alveolar artery.

☐ **C** The middle meningeal artery.

☐ **D** The deep temporal artery.

☐ **E** The lingual artery.

1.8

The lacrimal gland is supplied by the zygomaticotemporal nerve (V2), which conveys parasympathetic secretomotor fibres to it via the lacrimal nerve from V1.

Postsynaptic parasympathetic and sympathetic fibres also supply the glands of the nasal cavity, palate and upper pharynx.

1.9 Answer: A, B, C, D

The maxillary artery is divided into three divisions, each division having five branches.

(1) Mandibular division – each branch leads to a bony foramen:
  – inferior alveolar artery – runs to the mandibular foramen to the mandibular teeth
  – middle meningeal artery – to foramen spinosum and runs deep to pterion
  – accessory meningeal – runs through foramen ovale with V3.
(2) Pterygoid division – each branch serves a muscle:
  – masseteric branch
  – medial and lateral pterygoid.
  – buccal
  – temporals – two deep temporal arteries.
(3) Pterygopalatine division – each branch is a terminal branch of the maxillary artery:
  – infraorbital artery – runs in infraorbital foramen with infraorbital branch of V2
  – posterior superior alveolar – to maxillary teeth
  – (long) sphenopalatine artery – to nasal cavity
  – pharyngeal branch
  – descending palatine – becomes the greater and lesser palatine arteries to the hard and soft palate, respectively.

1.10 **The parotid gland:**

☐ **A** Receives parasympathetic innervation from fibres which synapse with axons that travel in the greater petrosal nerve.

☐ **B** Surrounds part of the maxillary nerve.

☐ **C** Empties into the mouth opposite the second mandibular molar tooth.

☐ **D** Is enclosed within a sheath.

☐ **E** Sensory innervation to the gland is provided by the auriculotemporal nerve.

1.11 **The maxillary sinus:**

☐ **A** Is the first sinus to develop.

☐ **B** Is supplied by the greater palatine nerve.

☐ **C** Is supplied by the lesser palatine nerve.

☐ **D** Is supplied by branches of the greater palatine artery.

☐ **E** Has a sphenopalatine ganglion that lies anterior to the posterior wall.

1.12 **Structures running through the parotid gland include:**

☐ **A** The facial nerve.

☐ **B** The auriculotemporal nerve.

☐ **C** The facial artery.

☐ **D** The external carotid artery.

☐ **E** The retromandibular vein.

1.10 Answer: all true

The *parotid duct* leaves the anterior border of the gland travelling horizontally until it reaches the anterior border of the masseter. It then turns medially to pierce the buccinator obliquely at a point corresponding to the maxillary third molar, and enters the oral cavity opposite the upper second molar.

Sensory innervation to the gland is provided by the great auricular nerve and to the surrounding capsular fascia by the auriculotemporal nerve.

1.11 Answer: A, B, D

The *maxillary sinus* is innervated by:

- branches of V2 – the greater palatine nerve
- branches of the infraorbital nerve.

Behind the posterior wall is the:

- pterygomaxillary fossa with the internal maxillary artery
- sphenopalatine ganglion
- vidian canal
- greater palatine nerve
- foramen rotundum.

The anterior wall has an infraorbital foramen located at the superior portion, with the infraorbital nerve running over the roof of the sinus and exiting through the foramen.

The roof is formed by the orbital floor and transsected by the course of the infraorbital nerve.

1.12 Answer: A, D, E

The *parotid gland* has the facial nerve, external carotid artery and retromandibular vein running through it.

Anatomy answers

1.13 **The tympanic nerve:**

☐ **A** Is given off at the jugular foramen from the glossopharyngeal.

☐ **B** Carries parasympathetic innervation to the parotid gland via the lesser petrosal nerve.

☐ **C** Synapses at the pterygopalatine ganglion.

☐ **D** Forms the tympanic plexus in the middle ear.

☐ **E** Carries parasympathetic innervation to the parotid gland via the greater petrosal nerve.

1.14 **The facial artery:**

☐ **A** Can be palpated as the artery crosses the mandible just anterior to the masseter muscle.

☐ **B** Lies superficial to zygomaticus major.

☐ **C** Gives off the superior labial branch.

☐ **D** Gives off the inferior labial branch.

☐ **E** Heads towards the inner canthus of the eye.

1.13　Answer: all true

The *tympanic nerve* is a branch of the glossopharyngeal nerve that exits the jugular foramen. It re-enters the skull through the inferior tympanic canaliculus and reaches the tympanic cavity where it forms a plexus in the middle-ear cavity. The nerve travels from this plexus through a canal and out into the middle cranial fossa adjacent to the exit of the greater petrosal nerve. It is here that the nerve becomes the lesser petrosal nerve. The *lesser petrosal nerve* exits the cranium via the foramen ovale and synapses in the otic ganglion.

The otic ganglion provides nerve fibres to the parotid gland. In the tympanic cavity it divides into branches, which form *the tympanic plexus* and are contained in grooves upon the surface of the promontory.

This plexus gives off:

• the lesser superficial petrosal nerve
• a branch to join the greater superficial petrosal nerve
• branches to the tympanic cavity.

1.14　Answer: A, C, D, E

The *facial artery* arises from the external carotid and winds to the inferior border of the mandible deep to the platysma. It crosses the mandible, buccinator and maxilla as it courses over the face to the medial angle of the eye. The facial artery lies deep to the zygomaticus major and levator labii superioris muscles. It eventually anastomoses with the ophthalmic artery.

Branches are:

• ascending palatine artery (a.)
• tonsillar branch
• submental a.
• superior labial a.
• inferior labial a.
• lateral nasal a.
• angular a.

1.15 **The mandibular nerve:**

- [ ] **A** Is a purely sensory nerve.
- [ ] **B** Innervates the tensor palatine.
- [ ] **C** Innervates the anterior belly of digastric.
- [ ] **D** Innervates the geniohyoid.
- [ ] **E** Exits through the foramen rotundum.

1.16 **The atlas:**

- [ ] **A** Allows a greater range of motion than normal vertebrae.
- [ ] **B** Has a spinous process.
- [ ] **C** Has a vertebral groove for the vertebral artery.
- [ ] **D** Has an odontoid process.
- [ ] **E** Has a superior articular facet.

1.17 **The lateral pterygoid muscle:**

- [ ] **A** Is attached to the greater wing of the sphenoid bone.
- [ ] **B** Is attached to the angle of the mandible.
- [ ] **C** Is attached to the capsule of the temporomandibular joint.
- [ ] **D** Is innervated by the mandibular nerve.
- [ ] **E** Has the inferior alveolar and lingual nerves related to its lower border.

1.15 Answer: B, C

The *mandibular nerve* exits the cranium by descending through the foramen ovale.

It supplies sensation to the lower third of the face and the tongue, floor of the mouth and jaw.

The motor root of the mandibular nerve innervates the *four muscles of mastication*: the mylohyoid, anterior belly of digastric, tensor tympani and tensor vali palatini. The geniohyoid is supplied by the ansa cervicalis.

1.16 Answer: A, C, D, E

The *atlas*:

- has no body
- has no spinous process
- is ring-like
- consists of an anterior arch, a posterior arch and two lateral masses.

Immediately behind each superior articular process is a groove that arches backward from the posterior end of the superior articular process. This groove represents the superior vertebral notch, and serves for the transmission of the vertebral artery; after ascending through the foramen in the transverse process, this winds around the lateral mass backward and medially; it also transmits the suboccipital nerve (first spinal nerve).

1.17 Answer: A, C, D, E

The *lateral pterygoid muscle* on each side is one of the muscles that act on the temporomandibular joint. It arises from two heads:

(1) Superior head: infratemporal surface of the greater wing of the sphenoid bone.
(2) Inferior head: lateral surface of the lateral pterygoid plate.

It passes superiorly, laterally and posteriorly to insert at two sites: the internal surface of the neck of the mandible and the intra-articular cartilage of the temporomandibular joint. It is innervated by the mandibular nerve (V3) by the lateral pterygoid nerve.

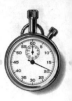

1.18   The parotid bed houses the deep part of the gland that fills the small space between the neck of the condyle of the mandible and the mastoid process. Other structures forming the floor of this space include:

A   The styloid process.

B   The styloglossus muscle.

C   The stylopharyngeus muscle.

D   The anterior belly of digastric.

E   The posterior belly of the digastric muscle.

1.19   Which of the following is true with regard to the sinuses of the brain?

A   The sigmoid sinus drains into the jugular vein.

B   The inferior sagittal sinus joins the great vein of Galen to form the straight sinus.

C   The cavernous sinus receives blood from the superior ophthalmic vein.

D   The cavernous sinus receives blood from the inferior ophthalmic vein.

E   The confluence of sinuses leads into the straight sinus.

1.20   Structures derived from the first branchial arch include:

A   The incus.

B   The maxillary artery.

C   The stylohyoid ligament.

D   The stylohyoid muscle.

E   The posterior third of the tongue.

1.18   Answer: A, C, E

The *structures forming the floor* of this space are:

- the styloid process
- the stylohyoid muscle
- the stylopharyngeus muscle
- the posterior belly of the digastric muscle.

1.19   Answer: A, B, C

The *great cerebral vein* is: formed by the union of the two internal cerebral veins – a short median trunk that curves backward and upward around the splenium of the corpus callosum and ends in the anterior extremity of the straight sinus.

The *cavernous sinus* receives the superior ophthalmic vein.

The *confluence of the sinuses* is usually found on one side (generally the right) of the internal occipital protuberance and the transverse sinus of the same side is derived from it.

1.20   Answer: A, B

The *second branchial arch* gives rise to the stylohyoid ligament and muscle, stapedius, posterior belly of digastric and the facial nerve.

The *third branchial arch* gives rise to the posterior third of the tongue, stylopharyngeus and the glossopharyngeal nerve.

The contents of the *first branchial arch* are as follows:

- Ectodermal and endodermal:
  - mucous membrane and glands of the anterior two-thirds of the tongue.
- Mesodermal:
  - muscles of mastication (chewing)
  - masseter
  - pterygoid muscles
  - temporalis muscles
  - mylohyoid muscle
  - digastric muscle, anterior belly
  - tensor palati muscle
  - tensor tympani muscle.

1.21   The basilar artery:

☐ A   Enters the cranium through the foramen magnum.

☐ B   Is formed by the union of two vertebral arteries.

☐ C   Supplies the lateral and third ventricles.

☐ D   Supplies the vermis through its superior cerebellar branch.

☐ E   Supplies the motor cortex.

1.22   The thyroid gland:

☐ A   Develops from the first and second pharyngeal arches.

☐ B   Contains cells derived from the fourth pharyngeal pouch.

☐ C   Is supplied mainly by the middle thyroid artery.

☐ D   Is covered by the pretracheal fascia.

☐ E   Has the recurrent laryngeal nerve ascending anteriorly.

1.23   The parathyroid glands:

☐ A   Are found on the posterior surface of the thyroid glands.

☐ B   Develop from the second and fourth pharyngeal pouch endoderm.

☐ C   May be confused with fat globules.

☐ D   Receive their blood supply from the middle thyroid arteries.

☐ E   Contain chief cells that have dark-staining nuclei.

1.24   The coeliac ganglion is:

☐ A   In front of L3.

☐ B   On the crura.

☐ C   Behind the pancreas.

☐ D   Behind the IVC.

☐ E   In front of the aorta.

1.21 Answer: B, C, D

The *basilar artery* is formed at the lower border of the pons. It supplies the posterior two-fifths of the cerebrum, part of the cerebellum and the brain stem.

The *middle cerebral artery* supplies the motor cortex.

1.22 Answer: A, B, D

The superior and inferior thyroid arteries mainly supply the *thyroid*.

The *recurrent laryngeal nerve* runs medial to the lateral lobe.

1.23 Answer: A, C, D, E

The inferior parathyroid glands and thymus develop from the third branchial pouch and the superior parathyroid glands from the fourth.

The main blood supply is from the superior and inferior thyroid arteries.

1.24 Answer: B, C, D, E

Usually, two *coeliac ganglia* are located on the abdominal aorta at the origin of the coeliac trunk in front of T12. Branches of the vagal trunks pass through the coeliac ganglion without synapsing.

1.25 The abdominal aorta:

- [ ] **A** Is separated posteriorly from the lumbar vertebrae by the azygos vein.
- [ ] **B** Is covered anteriorly by the left renal vein.
- [ ] **C** Is covered anteriorly by branches of the coeliac artery.
- [ ] **D** The azygos vein lies to its right.
- [ ] **E** The ascending part of the duodenum is on its left side.

1.26 The splenic artery:

- [ ] **A** Is accompanied by the vein that lies above it.
- [ ] **B** Crosses in front of the upper part of the left kidney.
- [ ] **C** Has the right gastroepiploic artery as a branch.
- [ ] **D** Has the arteria pancreatica magna as a branch.
- [ ] **E** Has branches passing to the greater curvature of the stomach between the layers of the gastrolienal ligament.

1.25   Answer: B, C, D

The *abdominal aorta* is covered:

- Anteriorly, by the lesser omentum and stomach, behind which are the branches of the coeliac artery and coeliac plexus; below these, by the lienal vein, pancreas, left renal vein, inferior part of the duodenum, mesentery and aortic plexus.
- Posteriorly, it is separated from the lumbar vertebrae and intervertebral fibrocartilages by the anterior longitudinal ligament and left lumbar veins.

On the right side, above it is in relation to the azygos vein, cisterna chyli, thoracic duct and right crus of the diaphragm.

On the left side are the left crus of the diaphragm, the left coeliac ganglion, the ascending part of the duodenum and some small intestine.

1.26   Answer: B, C, D, E

The *splenic artery* is the largest branch of the coeliac artery and passes along the upper border of the pancreas, accompanied by the vein, which lies below it. It crosses in front of the upper part of the left kidney, and, on arriving near the spleen, divides into branches:

- Some of these enter the hilus of that organ between the two layers of the phrenicolienal ligament to be distributed to the tissues of the spleen.
- Some are given to the pancreas.
- Others pass to the greater curvature of the stomach between the layers of the gastrolienal ligament.

  Its branches are:

  - the arteria pancreatica magna
  - the short gastric
  - the left gastroepiploic.

1.27 **The spleen:**

- ☐ **A** Contains malpighian bodies.
- ☐ **B** Is invested in a single coat.
- ☐ **C** Develops from the dorsal mesogastrium.
- ☐ **D** Has a convex gastric surface.
- ☐ **E** Is intraperitoneal.

1.28 **In the male, the superficial perineal space contains:**

- ☐ **A** The superficial perineal muscles.
- ☐ **B** The contents of the scrotum.
- ☐ **C** The membranous urethra.
- ☐ **D** The bulbourethral glands.
- ☐ **E** The pudendal nerves.

1.29 **All of the following paranasal sinuses drain into the middle meatus EXCEPT:**

- ☐ **A** The anterior ethmoid.
- ☐ **B** The maxillary.
- ☐ **C** The frontal.
- ☐ **D** The sphenoid.
- ☐ **E** The posterior ethmoid.

1.27 Answer: A, C, E

The *spleen* appears about week 5 as a localized thickening of the mesoderm in the dorsal mesogastrium above the tail of the pancreas. (Malpighian bodies or lymphatic nodules are local expansions or hyperplasia of the adenoid tissue, of which the external coat of the smaller arteries of the spleen is formed.)

Two coats invest the spleen: an external serous and an internal fibroelastic coat.

The gastric surface is concave and contacts the posterior wall of the stomach.

The spleen is almost entirely surrounded by peritoneum, which is firmly adherent to its capsule.

1.28 Answer: A, B, E

The contents of the *superficial perineal space* are:

- the root of the penis and the muscles associated with it
- the contents of the scrotum
- the proximal part of the spongy urethra
- the superficial perineal muscles
- the branches of the internal pudendal vessels
- the pudendal nerves.

1.29 Answer: D, E

The space under the middle turbinate is termed the 'middle meatus' into which the anterior ethmoids, frontal sinus and maxillary sinus drain.

The posterior ethmoid cells drain into the superior meatus.

The sphenoid drains into the space between the superior turbinate, the septum and the sphenoid sinus front wall (the sphenoethmoid recess).

1.30   **Ureters:**

☐ **A** Are retroperitoneal.

☐ **B** Have a ductus deferens that is superior and anterior to the ureter.

☐ **C** Pass directly inferior to the uterine artery as they pass over the pelvis to enter the bladder.

☐ **D** Are supplied by sympathetic autonomic nerves T11–L1.

☐ **E** Pass obliquely into the posterior bladder wall.

1.31   **The bladder:**

☐ **A** Has venous drainage to the vesicular venous plexus.

☐ **B** Has lymphatics that go primarily to both external and internal iliac nodes.

☐ **C** Has the urachus coming off its apex.

☐ **D** Is supplied by the superior and inferior vesical arteries only.

☐ **E** Has a rough, loosely associated surface throughout.

1.32   **The bony pelvis:**

☐ **A** Is android (wedge) shaped in males.

☐ **B** Is oval shaped in males.

☐ **C** Is oriented so that the urogenital diaphragm, connected to the ischiopubic rami, is in a horizontal position.

☐ **D** Has the pelvic diaphragm forming the inferior border.

☐ **E** Has sciatic notches that are wider and shallower in females.

1.30 Answer: all true

The course of the ureter is as follows:

- It passes along the medial part of the psoas behind but adherent to the peritoneum
- It crosses the bifurcation of the common iliac arteries anterior to the sacro-iliac joint
- At the ischial spine it passes forwards and medially to enter the bladder obliquely

In the female the uterine artery crosses the ureters anteriorly before the ureter enters the bladder. The uterine artery crosses the ureters superiorly. In the male the ureter is crossed superficially near its termination by the vas deferans (remember 'water under the bridge').

1.31 Answer: A, B, C

The trigone is smooth with tightly adherent muscle.

The arteries supplying the *bladder* are the superior, middle and inferior vesical arteries, derived from the anterior trunk of the hypogastric.

The obturator and inferior gluteal arteries also supply small visceral branches to the bladder, and in the female additional branches are derived from the uterine and vaginal arteries.

1.32 Answer: A, C, D, E

Compared with the male, the following apply to the female pelvis:

- It is oval shaped.
- The ilia are less sloped, and the anterior iliac spines more widely separated – hence the greater lateral prominence of the hips.
- The obturator foramina are triangular in shape and smaller in size.
- The sciatic notches are wider and shallower, and the spines of the ischia project less inward.
- The acetabula are smaller and face more distinctly forward.
- The ischial tuberosities and the acetabula are wider apart.
- The pubic symphysis is less deep, and the pubic arch is wider and more rounded.

1.33 **The pancreas:**

☐ **A** Lies anterior to the kidney.

☐ **B** Has a superior mesenteric artery that passes behind the uncinate process.

☐ **C** Has a junction of the splenic and superior mesenteric veins that lies behind the gland.

☐ **D** Is pierced by the superior colic artery.

☐ **E** Has a posterior surface in relation with the IVC.

1.34 **In the urethra:**

☐ **A** The prostatic part is the widest.

☐ **B** Rupture of the spongy part (in the bulb) is common in straddle injuries.

☐ **C** The membranous part passes through the external sphincter.

☐ **D** The spongy and membranous parts are supplied by the external pudendal artery.

☐ **E** Lymphatic drainage is mainly to the superficial inguinal nodes.

1.33   Answer: A, C, E

The right side of the pancreas is in contact with the transverse colon anteriorly.

The lower part of the right half, below the transverse colon, is covered by peritoneum continuous with the inferior layer of the transverse mesocolon and in contact with the small intestine.

The superior mesenteric artery passes down in front of the left half, across the uncinate process; the superior mesenteric vein runs upward on the right side of the artery and, behind the neck, joining with the splenic vein to form the portal vein.

The posterior surface is in relation with:

- the IVC
- the common bile duct
- the renal veins
- the right crus of the diaphragm
- the aorta.

1.34   Answer: A, B, C

The *internal pudendal artery* supplies the spongy and membranous parts.

Lymphatic drainage is mainly to the internal iliac lymph nodes.

1.35 Which of the following are true with regard to the thoracic diaphragm?

☐ A The sternocostal triangle is a gap in part of the diaphragm.

☐ B The sternocostal triangle transmits the superior epigastric artery.

☐ C The costal part of the diaphragm arises from the surface of the lower six costal cartilages and ribs.

☐ D The nerve supply to the peripheral part of the diaphragm is by way of the thoracoabdominal nerves.

☐ E The costal part of the diaphragm raises and everts the costal margin.

1.36 Which of the following are true with regard to the suprarenal glands?

☐ A The anterior relationship of the right suprarenal gland includes the liver, IVC and peritoneum.

☐ B The splenic artery crosses in front of the left suprarenal gland.

☐ C There are multiple suprarenal arteries that arise from the phrenic artery.

☐ D The suprarenal glands have a nerve supply from the coeliac plexus along with lumbar and thoracic splanchnic nerves.

☐ E The right suprarenal vein enters the IVC directly.

1.35 Answer: all true

The *diaphragm* is divided into three parts:

(1) The sternal part arises from the back of the xiphoid and descends to the central tendon.
(2) The costal part arises from the inner surface of the lowermost six costal cartilages and ribs. During contraction it raises and everts the costal margin. On each side, a small gap known as the *sternocostal triangle* is present between the sternal and costal parts. It transmits the superior epigastric vessels and some lymphatics, and it may be the site of a diaphragmatic hernia.
(3) The lumbar part arises from the bodies of lumbar vertebrae in the form of two fibrous arches:
    – medial lumbocostal arch (medial arcuate ligament)
    – lateral lumbocostal arch (lateral arcuate ligament).

The phrenic nerve is the main nerve supply of the diaphragm, but branches of the thoracoabdominal nerves also supply the peripheral portions.

1.36 Answer: all true

The *suprarenal glands* lie on the superomedial aspect of the kidney.

The right gland: lies behind and against the diaphragm and in front contacts the liver, IVC and peritoneum.

The left gland relates behind to the diaphragm and in front to the pancreas and the peritoneum of the lesser sac. The splenic artery crosses the suprarenal gland anteriorly.

Blood supply includes:

- multiple suprarenal arteries that arise from the phrenic artery
- a middle suprarenal artery arising from the aorta
- inferior suprarenal arteries that arise from the renal arteries.

The left suprarenal vein drains into the left renal vein and the right suprarenal vein into the IVC.

1.37 **Which of the following are true with regard to the anal triangle?**

- [ ] **A** The anal triangle is posterior to a transverse line joining the anterior ends of the ischial tuberosities.
- [ ] **B** The front boundary of the ischiorectal fossa is the posterior margin of the urogenital diaphragm.
- [ ] **C** The ischiorectal fossa contains the superior rectal vessel and nerves.
- [ ] **D** The ischiorectal fossa contains a branch of the posterior cutaneous nerve.
- [ ] **E** The ischiorectal fossa on either side communicates with the other behind the anal canal.

1.38 **The middle meningeal artery:**

- [ ] **A** Enters the skull through the foramen spinosum.
- [ ] **B** Supplies the dura mater and calvaria.
- [ ] **C** Has a posterior branch that is commonly torn in fractures of the pterion.
- [ ] **D** Produces a lucid interval after the occurrence of an extradural haemorrhage.
- [ ] **E** Has an anterior branch that crosses the lesser wing of the sphenoid.

1.37   Answer: A, B, D, E

The *anal triangle* is bounded in front by the posterior edge of the urogenital diaphragm and laterally by the sacrotuberous ligaments.

The *ischiorectal fossa* lies above the skin of the anal triangle and below the pelvic diaphragm. The inferior fascia of the pelvic diaphragm and the sphincter ani externus forms the superomedial wall of the ischial rectal fossa.

The front boundary of the ischiorectal fossa is the posterior margin of the urogenital diaphragm. The ischiorectal fossa on either side communicates with the other behind the anal canal.

The ischiorectal fossa contains:

- ischiorectal fat pad
- internal pudendal vessels
- pudendal nerve
- inferior rectal vessels and nerves
- a branch of the posterior femoral cutaneous nerve.

1.38   Answer: A, B, D

The *middle meningeal artery* ascends between the two roots of the auriculotemporal nerve to the foramen spinosum of the sphenoid bone, through which it enters the cranium; it then runs forwards in a groove on the great wing of the sphenoid bone, and divides into two branches – anterior and posterior.

The anterior branch crosses the great wing of the sphenoid, reaches the groove in the parietal bone and divides into branches that spread out between the dura mater and the internal surface of the cranium, some passing upwards as far as the vertex and others backwards to the occipital region.

The posterior branch divides into branches that supply the posterior part of the dura mater and cranium.

The branches of the middle meningeal artery are distributed partly to the dura mater, but chiefly to the bones; they anastomose with the arteries of the opposite side, and with the anterior and posterior meningeal arteries.

1.39 **In thyroidectomy:**

☐ **A** The inferior thyroid artery lies posterior to the carotid sheath.

☐ **B** The recurrent laryngeal nerve (RLN) usually runs superficial to the inferior thyroid artery.

☐ **C** Damage to the external laryngeal nerve causes loss of voice in the upper half-octave.

☐ **D** The right RLN is more vulnerable to trauma.

☐ **E** Voice hoarseness after thyroidectomy may be caused by oedema.

1.40 **With regard to the nerve supply to the thyroid:**

☐ **A** The internal branch of the superior laryngeal nerve (SLN) is sensory.

☐ **B** The left RLN is more vulnerable to disease/traumatic injury.

☐ **C** The external branch of the SLN innervates most laryngeal muscles above the vocal cords/folds.

☐ **D** The SLNs lie in close proximity to the superior thyroid artery.

☐ **E** The SLN does not supply the tongue.

1.39   Answer: A, C, E

After it branches off the vagus nerve, the left RLN loops around the aortic arch in the chest cavity and then courses back into the neck. This long course makes it at higher risk for injury compared with the shorter course of the right RLN which does not run through the chest cavity. At the lower part of the neck, the right recurrent laryngeal nerve crosses obliquely behind the inferior thyroid artery.

1.40   Answer: A, B, D

The *thyroid gland* receives its innervation primarily by the SLNs and the RLNs.

The posterior lateral portions of each lobe of the thyroid gland lie in extremely close proximity to each RLN.

The SLNs lie in close proximity to the superior thyroid artery and bifurcate into the internal and external branches.

The internal branch of the SLN is sensory and supplies sensation to the larynx above the level of the vocal folds.

The SLN also has branches to the base of the tongue.

The external branch of the SLN innervates the cricothyroid muscles, which tense the vocal folds.

On the right, the RLN exits the right vagus nerve and loops under the right subclavian vein, travels through the tracheo-oesophageal groove and pierces the cricothyroid membrane posteriorly.

Conversely, the left RLN loops around the aorta and courses along the tracheo-oesophageal groove, entering the larynx through the posterior cricothyroid membrane.

As a result of its longer course, the left RLN is more vulnerable to disease and traumatic injury than the right RLN.

The RLNs supply motor innervation to the intrinsic laryngeal muscles. These muscles assist in changing the position of the cricoid, arytenoid and thyroid cartilages, thus affecting both the tension and the length of the vocal folds. The RLN also supplies sensory innervation to the larynx below the level of the vocal folds.

1.41   **With regard to the facial nerve (cranial nerve VII):**

☐ **A** A lesion of the zygomatic branch may result in corneal ulceration.

☐ **B** The cervical branch supplies the platysma.

☐ **C** Lesions near the stylomastoid foramen result in loss of motor function only.

☐ **D** Descent is through the anterior wall of the middle ear.

☐ **E** The lingual nerve supplies taste to the soft palate.

1.42   **In the nasal cavity:**

☐ **A** The nasolacrimal duct opens into the middle meatus.

☐ **B** Septal haematoma may lead to a saddle-type nasal deformity

☐ **C** The nerve supply of the posteroinferior nasal mucosa arises from the maxillary nerve.

☐ **D** The superior concha is the longest of the nasal conchae.

☐ **E** Infections of the nasal cavity may spread to the anterior cranial fossa.

☐ **F** Atherosclerosis of the greater nasal arteries may cause epistaxis.

1.41   Answer: A, B, C

On the medial wall of the *tympanic cavity*, there is a rounded promontory (formed by the first turn of the cochlea).

Fibres of the facial and glossopharyngeal nerves form the tympanic plexus of nerves, lying on the promontory.

After exiting the stylomastoid foramen the *facial nerve* gives off branches to the posterior belly of digastric and the stylohyoid, as well as an auricular branch that supplies the occipitalis.

Within the parotid gland, the facial nerve breaks up into temporal, zygomatic, buccal, mandibular and cervical branches. These supply the *muscles of facial expression*, platysma, frontalis and buccinator.

Branches of the *lingual nerve* supply:

- the sublingual gland
- the mucous membrane of the mouth
- the gums
- the mucous membrane of the anterior two-thirds of the tongue.

The chordae tympani supply:

- taste to the soft palate
- the anterior two-thirds of the tongue.

1.42   Answer: B, C, E, F

The arterial supply to the *nasal fossa* is complex and involves branches from both the external (ECA) and internal (ICA) carotid arteries.

The ECA contributes most of its supply via the internal maxillary (sphenopalatine and greater palatine branches) and facial arteries.

The ophthalmic artery, usually a branch of the ICA, can supply the nasal fossa via the anterior and posterior ethmoidal arteries.

The sphenopalatine artery serves as the major supply to the nasal fossa via the lateral and medial branches.

The lateral branches supply the inferior, middle and superior turbinates.

The medial or septal branches supply the nasal septum.

The inferior nasal concha is the largest of the three.

The nasolacrimal duct drains into the inferior meatus.

Anatomy answers

1.43   Of the foramina:

- [ ] **A** Foramen magnum contains the medulla oblongata.
- [ ] **B** Foramen ovale contains the mandibular nerve.
- [ ] **C** Foramen lacerum contains the ICA.
- [ ] **D** Foramen magnum contains the spinal roots of cranial nerve XI.
- [ ] **E** Foramen spinosum contains the maxillary nerve.

1.44   Cerebrospinal fluid (CSF):

- [ ] **A** Has its total volume replaced two to three times in 24 hours.
- [ ] **B** Passes to the third ventricle via the cerebral aqueduct.
- [ ] **C** Provides nutrition for glial cells.
- [ ] **D** Gains access to the blood mainly through the arachnoid villi.
- [ ] **E** May be normal on lumbar puncture in bacterial meningitis.

1.45   The scalp:

- [ ] **A** Derives its blood supply from both internal and external branches of the carotid artery.
- [ ] **B** Is supplied by spinal cutaneous nerves C2 and C3.
- [ ] **C** Has arteries that run deep to the epicranial aponeurosis.
- [ ] **D** Contains no lymph nodes.
- [ ] **E** Has an aponeurosis layer that is injured in gaping scalp lacerations.

1.43   Answer: A, B, C, D

Foramen rotundum contains the maxillary nerve.

Foramen spinosum contains the middle meningeal artery.

1.44   Answer: B, C, D, E

CSF formed in the lateral ventricles escapes via the foramen of Monro into the third ventricle and, thence, via the aqueduct into the fourth ventricle.

From the fourth ventricle the fluid travels into the subarachnoid spaces through the median foramen of Magendie and the two lateral foramina of Luschka.

The main route by which CSF gains access to the blood is through the arachnoid villi, which are microscopic projections of pia arachnoid mater that extend into venous channels, providing CSF–vascular interfaces. Aggregations of villi, which are visible macroscopically, are referred to as arachnoid granulations.

The rate of formation is about 0.35 ml/min or 500 ml/day – a rate that replaces the total volume of CSF about two to three times in 24 hours.

The normal range for glucose content in the CSF is at least 60–70% of the blood glucose level but levels may be slightly increased if the person has just eaten.

1.45   Answer: A, B, D, E

The part of the scalp anterior to the auricles drains to the parotid, submandibular and deep cervical lymph nodes.

The posterior part of the scalp drains to the posterior auricular (mastoid) and occipital lymph nodes.

The scalp has a rich vascular supply. The blood vessels traverse the connective tissue layer, and receive vascular contribution from the internal and external carotid arteries. The blood vessels anastomose freely in the scalp.

From the midline anteriorly, the arteries present as follows: supratrochlear, supraorbital, superficial temporal, posterior auricular and occipital.

1.46   In the sinuses:

☐ A   The roof of the frontal sinus may form the floor of the anterior cranial fossa.

☐ B   The ethmoid sinuses are most prone to infection.

☐ C   Optic neuritis may result from infection of the maxillary sinuses.

☐ D   The frontal sinuses are innervated by branches of the supraorbital nerves.

☐ E   Nasal polyps most commonly arise from the maxillary sinuses.

1.47   In the pharynx:

☐ A   Tonsillar pain may be referred to the ear via branches of the glossopharyngeal nerve.

☐ B   The external palatine vein is usually the main source of haemorrhage after tonsillectomy.

☐ C   Lymph from the palatine tonsil drains to the inferior deep cervical nodes.

☐ D   Recurrent thyroiditis may be caused by a sinus tract from the piriform recess.

☐ E   The anterior part of Waldeyer's ring is formed by the palatine tonsils.

1.48   The pituitary gland:

☐ A   Is extradural.

☐ B   Could produce a tumour that can cause junctional scotoma.

☐ C   Is ectodermal in origin.

☐ D   Lies above the diaphragma sellae.

☐ E   Lies medial to the cavernous sinuses.

1.49   The cavernous sinus:

☐ A   On the right and left is connected by the circular sinus.

☐ B   Is formed between layers of dura mater.

☐ C   Receives blood from the middle cerebral vein.

☐ D   Can produce thrombosis (cavernous sinus thrombosis or CST) that is usually an early complication of an infection of the central face or paranasal sinuses.

☐ E   Empties into the inferior petrosal sinuses, which contain valves.

1.46   Answer: A, C, D

The *sinus* that is most commonly the site of infection is the maxillary sinus.

The ethmoid sinuses are situated between the eye and the nose, and are commonly infected in children. Most nasal polyps originate from the ethmoid sinuses.

The optic nerve may be involved when there is a breach of the thin wall that separates the optic wall from the paranasal sinuses.

1.47   Answer: A, B, C, D

The *palatine tonsils* are two prominent masses situated on either side between the palatoglossal and palatopharyngeal arches.

The lymphatic vessels pass to the deep cervical glands.

1.48   Answer: B, C, E

The *pituitary gland* is enclosed by the dura and lies below the diaphragm sellae.

1.49   Answer: A, B, C

The *cavernous sinuses* receive venous blood from the facial veins (via the superior and inferior ophthalmic veins) as well as the sphenoid and middle cerebral veins.

They, in turn, empty into the inferior petrosal sinuses, and then into the internal jugular veins and the sigmoid sinuses via the superior petrosal sinuses.

This network of veins contains no valves; blood can flow in any direction depending on the prevailing pressure gradients.

The right and left cavernous sinuses are connected both anteriorly and posteriorly via the circular sinus.

Cavernous sinus thrombosis is usually a late complication of an infection of the central face or paranasal sinuses.

1.50 **The transpyloric line:**

- [ ] **A** Bisects the line joining the angle of Louis to the pubic symphysis.
- [ ] **B** Passes through the body of the pancreas.
- [ ] **C** Passes through the fundus of the gallbladder.
- [ ] **D** Passes through the hila of the kidneys.
- [ ] **E** Is the origin of the superior mesenteric artery.

1.51 **In lymph drainage from the bladder:**

- [ ] **A** The superior part drains mainly to the external iliac nodes.
- [ ] **B** The inferior part drains mainly to the external iliac nodes.
- [ ] **C** The neck of the bladder drains to the common iliac nodes.
- [ ] **D** The superior part drains mainly to the internal iliac nodes.
- [ ] **E** The inferior part drains to the superficial inguinal nodes.

1.52 **Blood supply of the ureters may be derived from:**

- [ ] **A** Renal arteries.
- [ ] **B** Common iliac arteries.
- [ ] **C** Vesical arteries.
- [ ] **D** Testicular arteries.
- [ ] **E** Internal iliac arteries.

1.50 Answer: C, D, E

The *transpyloric line* is an imaginary horizontal line, half the distance between the jugular notch and the pubic symphysis.

Structures lying on this plane include:

- the pylorus
- the fundus of the gallbladder
- the origin of the superior mesenteric artery
- the duodenojejunal junction
- the neck of the pancreas
- the hila of the kidneys
- the vertebra L1
- the formation of the portal vein
- the ninth costal cartilages.

1.51 Answer: A, C

Part of *bladder*	Lymph nodes:
Superior	External iliac nodes
Inferior	Internal iliac nodes
Neck	Sacral or common iliac nodes.

1.52 Answer: all true

The arterial supply of the *ureters* varies according to the individual and also along the length of the ureters.

Branches may be received from all of the following:

- renal arteries
- abdominal aorta
- common iliac arteries
- testicular/ovarian arteries
- internal iliac arteries
- vesical/uterine arteries.

1.53 Loss of sensation over the superior medial part of the thigh and root of the penis, and atrophy of the left testis after left inguinal hernia repair, may indicate damage to the:

- [ ] **A** Ilioinguinal nerve.
- [ ] **B** Genitofemoral nerve.
- [ ] **C** Iliohypogastric nerve.
- [ ] **D** Testicular artery.
- [ ] **E** Cremasteric artery.

1.54 The supply to the scrotum is from the:

- [ ] **A** External pudendal artery.
- [ ] **B** Internal pudendal artery.
- [ ] **C** Inferior epigastric artery.
- [ ] **D** Femoral artery.
- [ ] **E** Testicular artery.

1.55 The dura is innervated by:

- [ ] **A** All three divisions of the trigeminal nerve.
- [ ] **B** The vagus nerve.
- [ ] **C** The hypoglossal nerve.
- [ ] **D** The facial nerve.
- [ ] **E** The sympathetic nervous system.

1.53 Answer: A, D, E

The major nerves in the inguinal region are the ilioinguinal, iliohypogastric and genitofemoral nerves. The ilioinguinal nerve traverses the inguinal canal near the external inguinal ring and provides unilateral sensory innervation to the pubic region and the upper portion of the scrotum or the labia majora. This is the nerve most commonly injured during open herniorrhaphy. The iliohypogastric nerve passes superior to the internal inguinal ring and provides sensory innervation to the skin superior to the pubis. The genital branch of the genitofemoral nerve travels within the spermatic cord to provide sensation to the scrotum and the medial thigh. The femoral branch of this nerve supplies sensation to the skin of the anterior thigh. Blood supply to the testes is from three vessels which anastomose in the spermatic cord and near the epididymis.

The testicular artery (from the aorta).

The cremasteric artery (a branch of the inferior epigastric artery).

The deferential artery (a branch of the superior vesical artery).

1.54 Answer: B, C, D

Blood supply to the *scrotum* is from the:

- internal pudendal artery – perineal branch forming posterior scrotal branches
- inferior epigastric artery – cremasteric branch
- femoral artery – external pudendal branches forming anterior scrotal branches.

1.55 Answer: A, B, C, E

The nerves of the *cranial dura mater* are from:

- the ophthalmic nerve
- the maxillary nerve
- the mandibular nerve
- the vagus
- the hypoglossal nerve
- the sympathetic nervous system.

1.56 **Which statement is true of the right atrioventricular (AV) valve?**

☐ **A** It is also called the mitral valve.

☐ **B** It is open during ventricular diastole.

☐ **C** It transmits oxygenated blood.

☐ **D** It is opened by the pull of the chordae tendinae.

☐ **E** It consists of two leaflets.

1.57 **The internal carotid artery:**

☐ **A** Has no branches in the neck.

☐ **B** Is separated from the internal jugular vein at the base of the skull by the facial nerve.

☐ **C** Ascends within the carotid sheath together with the vagus nerve and the internal jugular vein.

☐ **D** Enters the cranium through the carotid canal in the membranous area of the petrous part of the temporal bone.

☐ **E** Gives rise to the ophthalmic artery.

1.58 **Secretory (motor) neurons to the lacrimal gland are derived from:**

☐ **A** The greater petrosal nerve.

☐ **B** The motor root of the mandibular nerve.

☐ **C** The lacrimal nerve.

☐ **D** The deep petrosal nerve.

☐ **E** The lesser petrosal nerve.

1.56   Answer: none of the above

Ventricular diastole is the period when the ventricles relax and fill with blood.

The tricuspid valve has three leaflets.

The mitral valve has two leaflets.

The chordae tendinae and the papillary muscles do not pull the AV valves open.

1.57   Answer: A, C, D, E

The *internal carotid artery* ascends within the carotid sheath together with the vagus nerve and the internal jugular vein.

At the base of the skull the glossopharyngeal, vagus, accessory, and hypoglossal nerves lie between the artery and the vein.

1.58   Answer: B, C, D, E

The *greater petrosal nerve* (an intracranial branch of the facial nerve) arises adjacent to the geniculate ganglion; it passes a short course in the bone and emerges, at the hiatus of the canal for the greater petrosal nerve, into the middle cranial fossa.

After passing forwards between the dura mater and the semilunar ganglion, it unites with the deep petrosal nerve (a sympathetic branch of the internal carotid plexus) to form the nerve of the pterygoid canal.

The greater petrosal nerve provides parasympathetic innervation to the lacrimal, nasal and palatine glands, and sensory to the soft palate.

1.59 Forward movement of the condyle of the mandible during wide opening of the jaws is accomplished by:

- [ ] **A** The anterior part of the temporalis muscle.
- [ ] **B** The lateral pterygoid muscle.
- [ ] **C** The masseter muscle.
- [ ] **D** The medial pterygoid muscle.
- [ ] **E** The mylohyoid.

1.60 Contents of the cavernous sinus include:

- [ ] **A** The abducens nerve (VI).
- [ ] **B** The third cranial nerve
- [ ] **C** Postganglionic sympathetic fibres.
- [ ] **D** The maxillary nerve (V2).
- [ ] **E** The mandibular nerve (V3).

1.61 The cavernous sinuses receive venous blood from:

- [ ] **A** The superior ophthalmic vein.
- [ ] **B** The inferior ophthalmic vein.
- [ ] **C** The sphenoid veins.
- [ ] **D** The middle cerebral veins.
- [ ] **E** The pterygoid plexus.

1.59   Answer: all true

The *lateral pterygoid* muscle is responsible for opening the jaw and drawing the mandible forward.

The anterior part of the *temporalis* muscle elevates the mandible, whereas the posterior part retracts it.

The *masseter* is a powerful chewing muscle that elevates the mandible.

The *medial pterygoid muscle* elevates the mandible and can help to move it forward.

However, when the mouth is open, the lateral pterygoid is the most important muscle for drawing the mandible forward.

1.60   Answer: A, B, C, D

Cavernous sinus contents:

Cavernous sinus of small veins/sinusoids

Internal carotid artery

Cranial nerve (CN) VI

CN III, IV, V1, V2

1.61   Answer: all true

The cavernous sinuses receive venous blood from the facial veins (via the superior and inferior ophthalmic veins) as well as the sphenoid and middle cerebral veins. They, in turn, empty into the inferior petrosal sinuses, then into the internal jugular veins and the sigmoid sinuses via the superior petrosal sinuses. The cavernous sinus also has anastomoses with Pterygoid venous plexus and this provides a pathway by which infection can spread from face to brain. This web of veins contains no valves; blood can flow in any direction depending on the prevailing pressure gradients.

1.62 The broad ligament of the uterus is a double layer of peritoneum that encloses all of the following EXCEPT:

☐ A The ureter.

☐ B The ovarian ligament.

☐ C The uterine tube.

☐ D The round ligament.

☐ E The uterine artery.

1.63 The constrictor muscles of the pharynx receive their motor nerve supply from:

☐ A The glossopharyngeal nerve.

☐ B The hypoglossal nerve.

☐ C The spinal accessory nerve.

☐ D The sympathetic trunk.

☐ E The vagus nerve.

1.64 Which of the following are not branches of the ophthalmic nerve?

☐ A Zygomatic nerve.

☐ B Frontal nerve.

☐ C Nasociliary nerve.

☐ D Lacrimal nerve.

☐ E Superior alveolar nerve.

1.62   Answer: A

The *uterine tube* is found in the upper free margin of the broad ligament and is connected to the root of the mesovarium by the mesosalpinx.

The *ovary* is attached to the posterior part of the broad ligament by the mesovarium.

The ovarian ligament is in the free margin of the mesovarium.

The uterine artery is near the root of the broad ligament.

1.63   Answer: A, D, E

The *vagus nerve* supplies:

(1) Motor innervation to the muscles of the larynx and pharynx, with the exception of stylopharyngeus (innervated by the *glossopharyngeal nerve*).
(2) Motor innervation to the palate muscles, with the exception of tensor veli palatini (V3 division of the trigeminal nerve).

The *glossopharyngeal nerve* provides the sensory innervation to the pharynx.

The *hypoglossal nerve* provides motor innervation to the muscles of the tongue.

The *accessory nerve* provides motor innervation to the trapezius and the sternocleidomastoid.

The pharyngeal plexus of nerves which is formed by CNX and CNIX nerves and by sympathetic branches from the superior cervical ganglion supply the pharynx.

1.64   Answer: A, E

The *zygomatic* and *superior alveolar* nerves are branches of the maxillary nerve.

1.65 **The trachea:**

- [ ] **A** Is lined by pseudo-stratified columnar epithelium.
- [ ] **B** Is separated from the manubrium by sternohyoid and sternothyroid muscles.
- [ ] **C** Receives blood from the inferior thyroid artery.
- [ ] **D** Is only 3 mm wide in the infant.
- [ ] **E** Becomes more superficial in the neck as it descends.

1.66 **The pretracheal fascia:**

- [ ] **A** Splits to enclose the thyroid gland.
- [ ] **B** Fuses with the carotid sheath.
- [ ] **C** Passes in front of the brachiocephalic veins.
- [ ] **D** Lies superficial to omohyoid.
- [ ] **E** Adheres to the isthmus of the thyroid gland and the second, third and fourth tracheal rings.

1.67 **With regard to gustation (taste):**

- [ ] **A** There are three basic taste sensations.
- [ ] **B** Taste buds are modified epithelial cells.
- [ ] **C** Taste buds are mostly found in vallate papillae.
- [ ] **D** Each taste bud consists of up to five spindle-shaped epithelial cells.
- [ ] **E** Each taste bud contains three different cell types.

1.65   Answer: A, B, C, D

The trachea becomes deeper as it descends in the neck.

1.66   Answer: A, B, D, E

The *pretracheal fascia* passes behind the brachiocephalic veins to blend with the adventitia of the arch of the aorta and the pericardium.

It adheres to the isthmus of the thyroid gland and the second, third and fourth tracheal rings.

It lies deep to the strap muscles.

1.67   Answer: B, C, E

There are four taste sensations – sweet, sour, salt and bitter.

Each *taste bud* has up to 50 spindle-shaped epithelial cells.

Each taste bud contains three different cell types – namely:

- supporting cells
- taste cells
- basal cells.

1.68 **With regard to muscles of the tympanic cavity:**

☐ **A** Tensor tympani originates from the tympanic tube.

☐ **B** Tensor tympani inserts into the incus.

☐ **C** Stapedius is innervated by the facial nerve.

☐ **D** Both tensor tympani and stapedius control tympanic membrane movement.

☐ **E** Stapedius lies within the facial canal.

1.69 **The suprascapular artery:**

☐ **A** Supplies muscles on the posterior scapula.

☐ **B** Is a branch of the thyrocervical trunk.

☐ **C** Passes posterior to the phrenic nerve.

☐ **D** Lies anterior to scalenus anterior.

☐ **E** Passes anterior to the brachial plexus.

1.70 **The third cranial nerve supplies:**

☐ **A** Lateral rectus.

☐ **B** Ciliary body.

☐ **C** Inferior oblique.

☐ **D** Medial rectus.

☐ **E** Superior oblique.

1.68   Answer: A, C, E

Stapedius lies within a small bony canal that communicates with the facial canal. It levers the footplate of the stapes and dampens the transmission of sound.

Tensor tympani pulls the eardrum inwards and pushes the footplate of the stapes into the vestibular window. This muscle inserts into the handle of the malleus and is innervated by the chorda tympani.

1.69   Answer: A, B, D, E

The *suprascapular artery* is a branch of the thyrocervical trunk on the subclavian artery.

It passes inferolaterally over:

- scalenus anterior
- the phrenic nerve
- the subclavian artery
- the brachial plexus.

It passes posterior to the scapula and supplies the muscles on its posterior aspect.

1.70   Answer: B, C, D

The *oculomotor nerve* forms anterior and inferior divisions on passing through the superior orbital fissure.

The superior division supplies:

- levator palpebrae superioris
- the superior rectus.

The inferior division supplies:

- the inferior rectus
- the medial rectus
- the inferior oblique
- the ciliary body.

1.71   With regard to the hand:

A   Dorsal interossei cause finger abduction.

B   Flexor digitorum superficialis (FDS) inserts into the distal phalanges.

C   Flexor digitorum profundus (FDP) inserts into the metacarpals.

D   The four lumbricals are supplied by the median nerve.

E   The lumbricals attach to the tendons of FDP.

1.72   The middle meningeal artery (MMA):

A   Is a branch of the maxillary artery.

B   Passes through foramen spinosum.

C   If damaged, may result in a subarachnoid haemorrhage.

D   Lies in the middle cranial fossa.

E   Passes through the foramen lacerum.

1.73   The umbilical artery:

A   Is a branch of the internal iliac artery.

B   Carries deoxygenated blood from the fetus.

C   If cannulated, may result in ischaemia of the gluteal region.

D   If unpaired, may be associated with congenital abnormalities.

E   Supplies the superior aspect of the urinary bladder in females.

1.74   Meckel's diverticulum:

A   Is a remnant of the vitello-intestinal duct.

B   Occurs in 0.2% of patients.

C   Is found on the anti-mesenteric border of the terminal ileum.

D   May contain ectopic colonic mucosa.

E   May present with intussusception.

1.71   Answer: A, E

Palmar interossei adduct, whereas dorsal *interossei* abduct the fingers.

The FDP inserts into the distal phalanges, whereas the FDS inserts into the middle phalanges.

Only the lateral two lumbricals are supplied by the median nerve.

1.72   Answer: A, B, D

The MMA passes through the foramen spinosum.

It divides into anterior and posterior divisions in the middle cranial fossa. Damage results in extradural haemorrhage.

1.73   Answer: all true

The paired *umbilical arteries* are branches of the internal iliac arteries and carry deoxygenated blood to the placenta.

If cannulated, blood supply to the inferior gluteal artery (another anterior branch of the internal iliac) may be interrupted.

1.74   Answer: A, C, D, E

Rule of twos:

(1) Occurs in 2% of patients, is 2 cm long and located 2 feet (0.6 m) from the ileocaecal junction.
(2) Usually an incidental finding at laparotomy but may result in rectal bleeding (caused by ectopic gastric mucosa), or umbilical discharge, small bowel volvulus or intussusception.

1.75   Hunter's canal:

☐ A   Contains the femoral artery.

☐ B   Contains the nerve to vastus lateralis.

☐ C   Contains the femoral nerve.

☐ D   Has a roof formed by sartorius.

☐ E   Is bordered medially by vastus medialis.

1.76   Hasselbach's triangle:

☐ A   Is bordered laterally by the inferior epigastric artery.

☐ B   Is bordered medially by rectus abdominis.

☐ C   Contains the obturator nerve and vessels.

☐ D   Is the site of direct inguinal herniation.

☐ E   Is bordered inferiorly by the inguinal ligament.

1.77   The jugular foramen:

☐ A   Is in the parietal bone.

☐ B   Transmits the glossopharyngeal nerve.

☐ C   Transmits the external jugular vein.

☐ D   Is closely related to the inferior petrosal sinus.

☐ E   Contains the superior ganglion of the vagus nerve.

1.75   Answer: A, D

Hunter's canal, also known as the adductor or subsartorial canal is bordered:

- laterally by vastus medialis
- medially by adductor longus and magnus.

Its roof is formed by sartorius.

It contains:

- the saphenous nerve
- the nerve to vastus medialis
- the femoral artery
- the femoral vein.

1.76   Answer: A, B, D, E

Also known as the *inguinal triangle*, Hasselbach's triangle is bordered:

- inferiorly by the inguinal ligament
- laterally by the inferior epigastric artery
- medially by the lateral edge of rectus abdominis.

Its floor is formed by the transversalis fascia.

It contains nothing.

1.77   Answer: B, D, E

The *jugular foramen* lies between the petrous temporal and occipital bones in the posterior cranial fossa.

It contains:

- the internal jugular vein (formed by the inferior petrosal and sigmoid sinuses)
- the glossopharyngeal and accessory nerves.

1.78   With regard to the foramina:

- [ ]   **A**   The frontal nerve enters the orbit through the superior orbital fissure.
- [ ]   **B**   The foramen rotundum contains the mandibular nerve.
- [ ]   **C**   The jugular foramen contains the vagus nerve.
- [ ]   **D**   The foramen magnum contains the vertebral arteries.
- [ ]   **E**   The foramen spinosum contains the maxillary nerve.

1.79   With regard to the sinuses:

- [ ]   **A**   The roof of the maxillary sinus is formed by the floor of the orbit.
- [ ]   **B**   The ethmoid sinuses are most prone to infection.
- [ ]   **C**   Infections of the nasal cavities may spread to the anterior cranial fossa through the cribiform plate.
- [ ]   **D**   The frontal sinuses are innervated by branches of the nasociliary nerves.
- [ ]   **E**   Nasal polyps most commonly arise from the ethmoid sinuses.

1.80   In the pharynx:

- [ ]   **A**   Tonsillar pain may be referred to the ear via branches of the glossopharyngeal nerve.
- [ ]   **B**   The external palatine vein is usually the main source of haemorrhage after tonsillectomy.
- [ ]   **C**   Lymph from the palatine tonsil drains to the inferior deep cervical nodes.
- [ ]   **D**   Recurrent thyroiditis may be caused by a sinus tract from the piriform recess.
- [ ]   **E**   The anterior part of Waldeyer's ring is formed by the palatine tonsils.

1.78 Answer: A, C, D

The *foramen spinosum* contains the middle meningeal artery and the meningeal branch of the mandibular nerve.

The jugular foramen contains the glossopharyngeal, vagus and acessory nerves as well as the internal jugular vein. The foramen rotundum contains the maxillary branch of the trigeminal nerve. The superior orbital fissure contains the frontal lacrimal and nasociliary branches of the trigeminal nerve, oculomotor, trochlear and abducent nerves as well as ophthalmic veins.

1.79 Answer: A, B, C and E

The *maxillary sinuses* are most commonly infected because their ostia are located high on the medial wall. Polyps most commonly arise from the ethmoid sinuses.

The frontal sinuses are innervated by branches of the supraorbital nerves (IV, VI).

1.80 Answer: A, B, D

The glossopharyngeal nerve (IX) supplies the middle ear and mucosal surface of the tympanic membrane via Jacobson's nerve and the tympanic plexus. Otalgia referred via the glossopharyngeal nerve arises from the oropharynx, including the tonsils and the base of tongue, nasopharynx and eustachian tube. The tonsils form part of a circular band of adenoid tissue that guards the opening into the digestive and respiratory tubes. The anterior part of the ring is formed by the *lingual tonsil* on the posterior part of the tongue; the lateral portions consist of the palatine tonsils and the tubular tonsils near the opening of the eustachian tubes, whereas the ring is completed behind by the pharyngeal tonsil on the posterior wall of the pharynx.

Anatomy answers

1.81 **With regard to the axilla:**

- A The first to fourth ribs form its medial wall.
- B Pectoralis major forms the lateral wall.
- C It contains part of the subclavian artery.
- D The subscapular artery is the largest branch of the axillary artery.
- E Hyperabduction syndrome may result in hand oedema.

1.82 **In the elbow:**

- A The medial epicondyle of the humerus is the origin for the flexors of the forearm.
- B The carrying angle is 10° more acute in men than in women.
- C The radial–ulnar bursa lies anterior to the supinator.
- D The ulnar nerve passes posterior to the lateral epicondyle.
- E The radial collateral ligament extends from the medial epicondyle of the humerus.

1.83 **The adductor canal:**

- A Contains the saphenous nerve.
- B Contains the nerve to vastus intermedius.
- C Contains the femoral vein.
- D Is bound medially by adductor longus.
- E Can be found in the thigh.

1.84 **Severance of the common peroneal nerve may result in:**

- A Foot drop.
- B Loss of sensation over the dorsum of the foot.
- C A high stepping gait.
- D Loss of sensation in the first interdigital cleft.
- E Loss of plantar flexion.

1.81 Answer: A, D, E

Pectoralis major forms the anterior wall of the axilla.

The subclavian artery becomes the axillary artery at the lateral border of the first rib.

1.82 Answer: A

The radial collateral ligament is attached, *above,* to a depression below the lateral epicondyle of the humerus; *below,* to the annular ligament, some of its most posterior fibres passing over that ligament, to be inserted into the lateral margin of the ulna.

The ulnar nerve passes posterior to the medial epicondyle.

The radial–ulnar bursa lies deep to the supinator.

1.83 Answer: A, C, E

The adductor canal (Hunter's canal) is an aponeurotic tunnel in the middle third of the thigh, extending from the apex of the femoral triangle to the opening in the adductor magnus. It is bounded, in front and laterally, by vastus medialis, behind by adductor longus and magnus, and medially by sartorius. The canal contains the femoral artery and vein, the saphenous nerve and the nerve to vastus medialis.

1.84 Answer: A, B, C, D

Injury to the common peroneal nerve commonly occurs where it winds lateral to the neck of the fibula. This would lead to partial or complete paralysis of the extensors and evertors of the foot (digital extensors, tibialis anterior and peronei) and also to loss of sensation in the lower part of the anterior surface of the limb.

1.85 **In the menisci:**

☐ **A** The lateral meniscus is more freely movable than the medial meniscus.

☐ **B** The lateral meniscus is typically C shaped.

☐ **C** The medial meniscus is firmly attached to the tibial collateral ligament.

☐ **D** Both are avascular apart from the periphery.

☐ **E** Tears confined to the anterior horn of the cartilage are unusual.

1.86 **Gluteus maximus:**

☐ **A** Originates from the internal surface of the ilium.

☐ **B** Inserts mainly into the iliotibial tract of the fascia lata.

☐ **C** Is a powerful extensor.

☐ **D** Is supplied by the superior gluteal nerve.

☐ **E** Is supplied by the inferior gluteal nerve.

1.87 **Which of the following are true about the muscles of the back?**

☐ **A** Latissimus dorsi arises from the spines of the lower six thoracic vertebrae, the lumbodorsal fascia and the iliac crest.

☐ **B** The thoracodorsal nerve supplies the latissimus dorsi.

☐ **C** The trapezius muscle is innervated by branches of the axillary nerve.

☐ **D** The latissimus dorsi inserts into the intertubercular groove of the humerus

☐ **E** The trapezius inserts into the anterior border of the clavicle.

1.88 **The long saphenous vein:**

☐ **A** Arises from the dorsal venous arch.

☐ **B** Passes posterior to the medial malleolus of the tibia.

☐ **C** Empties into the femoral vein.

☐ **D** Is accompanied by the sural nerve.

☐ **E** Has the superficial epigastric as one of its tributaries.

1.85   Answer: A, C, D, E

The lateral meniscus is typically circular.

1.86   Answer: B, C, E

Gluteus maximus originates from the external surface of the ilium above the posterior gluteal line, from the adjoining parts of the sacrum and coccyx, and from the sacrotuberous ligament. It inserts mainly into the iliotibial tract of the fascia lata, and to a lesser extent into the gluteal tuberosity of the femur. Thus, its main action is as a powerful extensor of the hip. Its insertion into the tibia through the iliotibial tract allows it to hyperextend the already extended knee joint; this is important in the maintenance of the standing position. It is supplied by the inferior gluteal nerve (L5, S1, S2).

1.87   Answer: A, B, D

The superficial muscles of the back include latissimus dorsi, trapezius, levator scapulae, rhomboid minor and rhomboid major.

Latissimus dorsi inserts into the intertubercular groove of the humerus and is supplied by the thoracodorsal nerve. The trapezius muscle arises from the spines of C7 and all the thoracic vertebrae, as well as from the superior nuchal line and external protuberance of the occipital bone. It inserts into the posterior border of the clavicle and the medial border of the acromion. It is innervated by the accessory nerve and third and fourth cervical nerves.

1.88   Answer: A, C, E

The long saphenous vein usually receives the superficial epigastric, superficial circumflex iliac and superficial external pudendal veins immediately before it enters the common femoral vein. The short saphenous vein is accompanied by the sural nerve on the lateral margin of Achilles' tendon.

1.89   The posterior cruciate ligament:

- [ ] **A** Inserts on the anterior intercondylar area of the tibia.
- [ ] **B** Attaches to the lateral side of the medial femoral condyle.
- [ ] **C** Is twice as strong as the anterior cruciate ligament.
- [ ] **D** Is usually injured as a result of a posterior force to the proximal tibia.
- [ ] **E** Attaches to the medial side of the lateral femoral condyle.

1.90   The anterior cruciate ligament:

- [ ] **A** Is intrasynovial.
- [ ] **B** Is intracapsular.
- [ ] **C** Is innervated by terminal branches of the tibial nerve.
- [ ] **D** Originates from the posteromedial aspect of the lateral femoral condyle.
- [ ] **E** Inserts on the tibia anterior and lateral to the medial intercondylar eminence.

1.91   Twisting injuries of the knee in athletes resulting in the unhappy triad of injuries involves:

- [ ] **A** Posterior cruciate.
- [ ] **B** Anterior cruciate.
- [ ] **C** Fibular collateral ligament.
- [ ] **D** Medial menisci.
- [ ] **E** Tibial collateral ligament.

1.92   The cubital fossa:

- [ ] **A** Is bound by pronator teres medially.
- [ ] **B** Is bound by brachialis laterally.
- [ ] **C** Is bound by supinator laterally.
- [ ] **D** Has the roof formed by the bicipital aponeurosis.
- [ ] **E** Is bound by biceps brachii medially.

| 1.89 | Answer: B, C, D |

The posterior cruciate ligament (PCL) inserts on the posterior intercondylar area of the tibia and attaches to the lateral side of the medial femoral condyle.

| 1.90 | Answer: B, C, D, E |

The cruciate ligaments are enclosed by a synovial envelope originating from the posterior aspect of the joint capsule, making them intra-articular but extrasynovial. The anterior cruciate ligament (ACL) runs posteriorly and upwards from its insertion on the central anterior position on the tibia to its origin on the posterior lateral wall of the intercondylar notch of the femur.

| 1.91 | Answer: B, D, E |

Unhappy triad of O'Donoghue: the combination of a medial collateral ligament tear, with tears of the meniscus and anterior cruciate ligament, is called 'the unhappy triad'.

| 1.92 | Answer: A, D |

The cubital fossa is bound by pronator teres medially; has the roof formed by the bicipital aponeurosis.

1.93 **The contents of the cubital fossa are:**

☐ **A** The commencement of the radial artery.

☐ **B** The biceps tendon.

☐ **C** The radial nerve.

☐ **D** The median nerve between the brachial artery and the brachioradialis tendon.

☐ **E** The median nerve between the brachial artery and the bicipital aponeurosis.

1.93   Answer: A, B

Pronator teres medially.

Brachioradialis laterally.

Brachialis and supinator muscles, which form the floor.

Bicipital aponeurosis and deep fascia, which form the roof.

The contents of the cubital fossa, from medial to lateral: median nerve, brachial artery, tendon of the biceps brachii and radial nerve (MATR).

Single best answer questions

1.94 Parasympathetic innervation to the parotid gland synapses in:

- [ ] **A** The trigeminal ganglion.
- [ ] **B** The superior cervical ganglion.
- [ ] **C** The otic ganglion.
- [ ] **D** The body of the parotid gland.
- [ ] **E** The ciliary ganglion.

1.95 Muscles important for abducting the vocal cords/folds include:

- [ ] **A** The cricothyroid.
- [ ] **B** The lateral cricoarytenoid.
- [ ] **C** The transverse arytenoids.
- [ ] **D** The thyroarytenoid.
- [ ] **E** The posterior cricoarytenoid.

1.96 The nasal lacrimal duct drains into:

- [ ] **A** The external auditory meatus.
- [ ] **B** The inferior meatus.
- [ ] **C** The middle meatus.
- [ ] **D** The superior meatus.
- [ ] **E** The internal auditory meatus.

1.97 Which of the following could cause an atrial septal defect?

- [ ] **A** Inadequate development of the foramen ovale.
- [ ] **B** Failure of the membranous part of the interventricular septum.
- [ ] **C** Inadequate development of conal ridges.
- [ ] **D** Excessive resorption of the septum primum.
- [ ] **E** Over-development of the septum secundum.

1.94 Answer: C

Parasympathetic secretory afferents to the parotid leave the inferior salivary nucleus with the glossopharyngeal nerve and travel via in the middle ear to synapse in the otic ganglion.

Postsynaptic fibres are distributed to the parotid by the auriculotemporal nerve.

1.95 Answer: E

The principal *muscle for vocal cord abduction* is the posterior cricoarytenoid (PCA) muscle.

The lateral cricoarytenoid (LCA) muscle, adducts the vocal fold and receives reinforcement from the transverse arytenoid muscles.

1.96 Answer: B

The *nasolacrimal duct* drains tears into the inferior meatus. (This explains why we develop nasal congestion when we cry.)

1.97 Answer: D

A patent *foramen ovale* usually results from abnormal resorption of the septum primum during the formation of the foramen secundum.

Ostium primum atrial septal defects are defects that result from a deficiency of the endocardial cushions and the atrioventricular septum.

The *septum primum* does not fuse with the endocardial cushions, resulting in a patent foramen primum.

1.98 Into which lymph nodes do lymphatic vessels from the anal canal, below the pectinate line, drain?

A   Para-aortic.

B   Superior mesenteric.

C   Internal iliac.

D   Superficial inguinal.

E   Inferior mesenteric.

1.98 Answer: D

The *anus* has two embryological origins:

(1) Inferior to pectinate line = ectoderm derivation.
(2) Superior to pectinate line = endoderm derivation.

The pectinate line joins the undersides of the anal valves (lower ends of the anal columns).

Lymphatic drainage is as follows:

- upper canal: internal iliac nodes
- lower canal: superficial inguinal nodes.

In addition to dividing the lymphatic drainage, the pectinate line also divides:

- the arterial supply
- the venous drainage
- the innervation of the anal canal.

The following are superior to the pectinate line:

- blood supply from the superior rectal artery
- blood draining via the superior rectal veins
- visceral innervation via the inferior hypogastric plexus.

The following are inferior to the pectinate line:

- inferior rectal arteries which are the main supply
- drainage via the middle and inferior rectal veins
- somatic innervation via the inferior rectal nerves.

1.99 Which of the following statements about the anal canal is true?

- [ ] **A** Internal haemorrhoids are painful to remove.
- [ ] **B** Lymphatic drainage inferior to the pectinate line is via the superficial inguinal nodes.
- [ ] **C** Anal mucosa superior to the pectinate line is derived from ectoderm.
- [ ] **D** Veins draining inferior to the pectinate line are tributaries of the portal system.
- [ ] **E** Inferior to the pectinate line, innervation is from the superior rectal nerve.

1.100 The prostate gland lies:

- [ ] **A** Within the urogenital diaphragm.
- [ ] **B** At the neck of the bladder and above the pelvic diaphragm.
- [ ] **C** At the neck of the bladder and below the pelvic diaphragm.
- [ ] **D** In the superficial perineal space.
- [ ] **E** In the rectovesical space.

1.99   Answer: B

The anal canal is comprised of two embryological regions. At the pectinate line, the hindgut (an endodermal derivative) meets the ectoderm. The pectinate line is demarcated by the distal end of the anal valves and a transition in epithelial types from the simple columnar epithelium of the gut to the stratified squamous epithelium of the epidermis occurs.

Inferior to pectinate line = ectoderm derivation.

Superior to pectinate line = endoderm derivation.

Anus has dual lymph drainage:

Below pectinate line =Superficial Inguinal Lymph nodes

Above pectinate line =Internal Iliac Lymphnodes

Arterial Supply: The superior rectal artery supplies the area superior to pectinate line, and the inferior rectal artery supplies the area inferior to the pectinate line. The middle rectal artery form anastamoses between the two parts.

Venous supply: Above the pectinate line, drainage is to superior rectal vein, below pectinate line, drainage is into inferior rectal veins.

Internal hemorrhoids are found within the anal columns superior to the pectinate line. Since the mucosa covering this part of the anal canal is derived from endoderm, it is insensitive to pain.

Nervous supply is via the following:

SOMATIC: Inferior rectal branches of pudendal nerve to the external sphincter, supplying Sensation to lower end of canal.

SYMPATHETIC: The pelvic plexus (preganglionic in L1/L2) which supplies the internal sphincter.

PARASYMPATHETIC: Pelvic splanchnics, which relax the internal sphincter and give afferent supply to upper part of canal.

1.100   Answer: B

The *prostate* is situated in the pelvic cavity:

- below the lower part of the symphysis pubis
- above the superior fascia of the urogenital diaphragm
- in front of the rectum.

1.101 The superior and inferior gluteal arteries arise from:

☐ **A** The internal iliac artery.

☐ **B** The superior rectal artery.

☐ **C** The common iliac artery.

☐ **D** The inferior epigastric artery.

☐ **E** The median sacral artery.

1.102 The internal iliac artery give rise to the following branches EXCEPT:

☐ **A** The superior gluteal.

☐ **B** The middle rectal.

☐ **C** The superior vesicle.

☐ **D** The internal pudendal.

☐ **E** The ovarian.

1.103 In the male, the membranous urethra:

☐ **A** Is within the prostate gland.

☐ **B** Starts at the trigone of the bladder.

☐ **C** is within the urogenital diaphragm.

☐ **D** Is within the corpus spongiosum.

☐ **E** Is called the ejaculatory duct.

1.104 After prostate surgery, your male patient is able to obtain an erection but cannot ejaculate. The nerve fibres that are most likely to have been damaged during surgery are:

☐ **A** The pelvic splanchnics.

☐ **B** The sympathetic fibres that synapse in the inferior hypogastric plexus.

☐ **C** The sympathetic fibres that synapse in the chain ganglia.

☐ **D** The somatic fibres in the sacral plexus.

☐ **E** The testicular plexus.

1.101 Answer: A

The superior and inferior gluteal arteries arise from the internal iliac artery.

1.102 Answer: E

Internal iliac artery branches:

Posterior division	Anterior division
Iliolumbar	Inferior gluteal
Lateral sacral	Middle rectal
Internal pudental	Uterine (females only)
Obturator	
Inferior vesical	
Inferior gluteal/superior gluteal	

1.103 Answer: C

The *membranous portion of the urethra* is the shortest, least dilatable and, with the exception of the external orifice, narrowest part of the canal. It extends downwards and forwards, with a slight anterior concavity, between the apex of the prostate and the bulb of the urethra. It perforates the urogenital diaphragm about 2.5 cm below and behind the pubic symphysis.

1.104 Answer: B

The nerve fibres most likely to have been damaged during surgery are the sympathetic fibres that synapse in the inferior hypogasthric plexus.

1.105 Most of the muscles that act on the shoulder girdle and upper limb joints are supplied by branches of the brachial plexus. Which of the following is NOT?

A Trapezius.

B Teres minor.

C Latissimus dorsi.

D Rhomboid major.

E Levator scapulae.

1.106 If you want to increase the muscle mass of latissimus dorsi, which of the following actions would you be most likely to perform?

A Depression of the scapula.

B Abduction of the arm.

C Extension of the arm.

D Flexion of the arm.

E Lateral rotation of the arm.

1.107 The true statement about the posterior compartment of the arm is that:

A It receives its motor supply from the median nerve.

B It contains a single elbow flexor.

C Its major artery is the radial artery.

D It contains the ulnar nerve in its distal part.

E Contains pronator teres.

1.108 The long head of the biceps brachii muscle arises from:

A The infraglenoid tubercle.

B The acromion process.

C The coracoid process.

D The clavicle.

E The supraglenoid tubercle.

1.105 Answer: A

Trapezius is innervated by branches of the ansa cervicalis and the spinal accessory nerve from the third and fourth cervical roots.

1.106 Answer: C

Latissimus dorsi extends, adducts and medially rotates the humerus at the shoulder; it draws the inferior angle of the scapula inferior and medial.

1.107 Answer: B

Functionally the brachioradialis is a forearm flexor but located in the posterior compartment of the arm. The median nerve is the principal nerve of the anterior compartment. The posterior compartment is supplied by the radial nerve. The brachial artery is the main arterial supply.

1.108 Answer: E

The long head of the biceps brachii muscle arises from the supragelnoid tubercle.

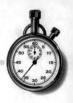

1.109 The distal attachment (insertion) of the triceps brachii muscle is:

☐ **A** The coronoid process of the ulna.

☐ **B** The olecranon process of the ulna.

☐ **C** The styloid process of the ulna.

☐ **D** The radial notch of the ulna.

☐ **E** The ulnar tuberosity.

1.110 The nerve most likely to be injured in fractures of the medial epicondyle is:

☐ **A** The radial.

☐ **B** The axillary.

☐ **C** The ulnar.

☐ **D** The median.

☐ **E** The musculocutaneous.

1.111 Which nerve is probably damaged if a patient CANNOT abduct the arm beyond 25°?

☐ **A** The axillary.

☐ **B** The radial.

☐ **C** The musculocutaneous.

☐ **D** The median.

☐ **E** The ulnar.

1.112 Which of the following muscles does NOT extend the wrist?

☐ **A** Extensor carpi radialis longus.

☐ **B** Extensor carpi radialis brevis.

☐ **C** Extensor carpi ulnaris.

☐ **D** Fxtensor digitorum.

☐ **E** Brachioradialis.

1.109 Answer: B

The distal attachment (insertion) of the triceps brachii muscle is the olecranon process of the ulna.

1.110 Answer: C

The ulnar nerve is in contact with bone as it courses posterior to the medial epicondyle where it is susceptible to injury from blunt trauma or fracture.

1.111 Answer: A

The deltoid is supplied by the axillary nerve.

1.112 Answer: E

Brachoradialis flexes the forearm.

1.113 After a cervical injury, a patient is unable to abduct the arm above the horizontal plane. This would be a result of an injury to:

A   The spinal accessory nerve.

B   The long thoracic nerve.

C   The axillary nerve.

D   All of the above.

E   None of the above.

1.114 A baby boy is born with hypospadias. Which of the following structures failed to fuse during development?

A   Anal folds.

B   Labioscrotal swellings.

C   Paramesonephric ducts.

D   Müllerian ducts.

E   None of the above.

1.115 The tetralogy of Fallot consists of all EXCEPT:

A   Pulmonary valve stenosis.

B   Ventricular septal defect.

C   Overriding aorta.

D   Hypertrophy of right ventricle.

E   Hypertrophy of left ventricle.

1.116 The foregut gives rise to all EXCEPT:

A   The lower respiratory system.

B   The pharynx.

C   The oesophagus.

D   The liver.

E   The jejunum.

1.113 Answer: A

The suprascapular nerve supplies supraspinatus responsible for initiating abduction. The deltoid then takes over (supplied by the axillary nerve). Since the serratus anterior and trapezius muscles are involved in rotating the scapula to allow abduction greater than 180 degrees damage to the long thoracic or the spinal accessory nerve can also impair abduction.

1.114 Answer: C

Hypospadias (occurs in 1 in 300 male births) is an abnormal opening of the urethra on to the ventral surface of the penis or scrotum, resulting from failure of the urethral folds to fuse.

Most cases occur on the distal penis or corona.

1.115 Answer: E

Typically *tetralogy of Fallot* consists of:

- pulmonary valve stenosis (the cusps of pulmonary valve are fused together to form a dome with a narrow central opening)
- ventricular septal defect
- overriding aorta
- hypertrophy of the right ventricle.

1.116 Answer: E

Foregut structures include:

- the pharynx
- the lower respiratory system
- the oesophagus
- the duodenum (proximal to the opening of the bile duct)
- the liver
- the pancreas
- the biliary apparatus.

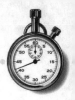

1.117 The most likely vessel to be damaged just behind the oesophagus and between the azygos vein is:

A   The hemiazygos vein.

B   The left bronchial vein.

C   The left pulmonary vein.

D   The superior vena cava.

E   The thoracic duct.

1.118 An obturator hernia that compresses the obturator nerve in the obturator canal may affect the function of all the following muscles EXCEPT:

A   Adductor brevis.

B   Adductor longus.

C   Gracilis.

D   Obturator externus.

E   Pectineus.

1.119 The following are typically not cyanotic congenital heart diseases EXCEPT for:

A   Patent ductus arteriosus.

B   Ventricular septal defect.

C   Atrial septal defect.

D   Tetralogy of Fallot.

E   Bicuspid aortic valve.

1.120 Which is NOT a branch of the external carotid artery?

A   Facial artery.

B   Superficial temporal artery.

C   Inferior thyroid artery.

D   Lingual.

E   Ascending pharyngeal artery.

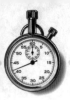

1.117   Answer: E

The *thoracic duct* is found directly behind the oesophagus in the posterior mediastinum, with the aorta to its left and the azygos vein to its right.

1.118   Answer: E

Pectineus is a muscle of the medial compartment of the thigh.

Most of the muscles in this compartment are adductors and medial rotators, innervated by the obturator nerve.

Pectineus is the exception in the medial compartment – the femoral nerve innervates it and it is a hip flexor.

1.119   Answer: D

Cyanotic heart disease includes:

- *tetralogy of Fallot*
- transposition of the great vessels
- total anomalous pulmonary venous return
- truncus arteriosus
- tricuspid atresia
- hypoplastic left heart syndrome.

1.120   Answer: C

The inferior thyroid artery is a branch of the thyrocervical trunk (which is a branch of the subclavian artery).

1.121 In the male, during a rectal examination, each of the structures below can be palpated (felt) EXCEPT for:

- [ ] A The prostate.
- [ ] B The sacrum.
- [ ] C The ductus deferens.
- [ ] D The coccyx.
- [ ] E The ischial tuberosity.

1.122 In the axilla, which is false?

- [ ] A The apical (subclavicular) lymph nodes in the apex of the axilla drain all the axillary lymph nodes.
- [ ] B The posterior cord of brachial plexus lies posterior to the first part of the axillary artery.
- [ ] C The tendon of latissimus dorsi lies anterior to the tendon of teres major.
- [ ] D The long thoracic nerve can be damaged in mastectomy.
- [ ] E Damage to the intercostobrachial nerve causes sensory loss over medial upper part of the arm.

1.123 Which of the following statements about head and neck anatomy is false?

- [ ] A The lymph from the upper lip drains to the submandibular nodes.
- [ ] B The facial nerve comes from the first pharyngeal arch.
- [ ] C Branches of the ophthalmic division of the trigeminal nerve supply the skin of the scalp as far back as the vertex.
- [ ] D The veins of the scalp are connected to both the diploic veins and the intracranial venous sinuses.
- [ ] E Unilateral cleft lip is a failure of the maxillary process to fuse with the medial nasal process.

1.124 With regard to the external jugular vein (EJV), which statement is false?

- [ ] A Arises from the retromandibular and posterior auricular veins.
- [ ] B Lies superficial to the sternocleidomastoid (SCM).
- [ ] C Pierces the deep fascia of the neck.
- [ ] D Drains blood from the scalp.
- [ ] E Receives the thoracic duct.

1.121   Answer: C

The *prostate* (lateral and posterior lobes) can be palpated on the anterior wall of the rectum (anterior and median lobes cannot be palpated).

Other structures that can be palpated include:

- the seminal vesicles of the bulb of the penis
- the ischial spines of the sacrospinous ligaments
- the ischial tuberosities of the sacrum and coccyx
- the ischioanal fossa wall of the rectum.

1.122   Answer: B

All three cords (lateral, medial, posterior) of the *brachial plexus* lie above and lateral to the first part of the axillary artery.

Latissimus dorsi, a large flat triangular muscle, sweeps over the lumbar region of the lower thorax. It ends as a flattened tendon about 7 cm long, anterior to teres major. Its nerve supply is the long thoracic nerve.

The long thoracic nerve can be damaged during an axillary dissection, causing winging of the scapula.

If an intercostobrachial nerve were damaged, patients would complain of medial upper arm numbness.

1.123   Answer: B

The *facial nerve* is derived from the second pharyngeal arch.

1.124   Answer: E

The EJV drains blood from the scalp and face.

It drains into the subclavian vein behind the medial end of the clavicle.

It pierces the deep fascia along with the anterior jugular vein, posterior to the clavicular head of SCM.

1.125 With regard to the thyroid gland, which statement is false?

☐ **A** It lies deep to sternohyoid.

☐ **B** It receives a middle thyroid artery from the external carotid artery.

☐ **C** The thyroglossal duct is closely related to the hyoid bone.

☐ **D** The isthmus lies over the second to third tracheal rings.

☐ **E** The pyramidal lobe is present in 50% of people.

1.126 The right lung contains the following number of segments:

☐ **A** Three.

☐ **B** Five.

☐ **C** Seven.

☐ **D** Ten.

☐ **E** Twelve.

1.127 The scaphoid articulates with all of the following EXCEPT:

☐ **A** Radius.

☐ **B** Lunate.

☐ **C** Capitate.

☐ **D** Triquetral.

☐ **E** Trapezium

1.128 The first part of the left subclavian artery is anterior to all EXCEPT:

☐ **A** The thoracic duct.

☐ **B** The oesophagus.

☐ **C** The left recurrent laryngeal nerve.

☐ **D** The left phrenic nerve.

☐ **E** The inferior cervical ganglion.

1.125   Answer: B

The *thyroid gland* lies between C5 and T1, and the isthmus is usually anterior to two to three tracheal rings.

It receives a superior thyroid artery from the external carotid artery and an inferior thyroid artery from the subclavian artery.

The middle thyroid vein drains into the internal jugular vein.

Fifty per cent have a pyramidal lobe that lies on the superior surface of the isthmus.

1.126   Answer: D

Each lung contains 10 bronchopulmonary segments.

1.127   Answer: D

The *scaphoid* articulates with the radius, lunate, capitate and trapezium.

1.128   Answer: D

The relations of the first part of the left subclavian artery are:

- In front, with the vagus, cardiac and phrenic nerves, which lie parallel with it, the left common carotid artery, left internal jugular and vertebral veins, and the start of the left brachio cephalic vein.
- Behind, with the oesophagus, thoracic duct, left recurrent nerve and inferior cervical ganglion of the sympathetic trunk.

1.129 With regard to the thoracic sympathetic chain, which statement is false?

- [ ] **A** The sympathetic outflow comes from T1–L2.
- [ ] **B** Pre-ganglionic fibres leave as white rami communicans to enter the sympathetic chain.
- [ ] **C** The sympathetic chain gives rise to the greater splanchnic nerve in the thorax.
- [ ] **D** The splanchnic nerves emerge from T12–L5.
- [ ] **E** The splanchnic nerves pass through the crura of the diaphragm.

1.130 With regard to the lateral ventricles, which statement is false?

- [ ] **A** The lateral ventricles consist of thee horns.
- [ ] **B** They connect to the third ventricle through the foramen of Monro.
- [ ] **C** The choroid plexus is located in the anterior and temporal horn.
- [ ] **D** The hippocampus forms the floor of the inferior horn.
- [ ] **E** The central part of the lateral ventricle also contains the choroid plexus.

1.131 All are true EXCEPT one. The subcostal nerve:

- [ ] **A** Passes behind the lateral arcuate ligament.
- [ ] **B** Passes through the transverses abdominis.
- [ ] **C** Does not supply the buttock.
- [ ] **D** Supplies part of rectus abdominis.
- [ ] **E** Lies below the vein and artery.

1.132 After surgical opening of the adductor canal, a patient experienced a loss of cutaneous sensation of the medial side of the leg. Which nerve was cut?

- [ ] **A** Ilioinguinal.
- [ ] **B** Femoral.
- [ ] **C** Obturator.
- [ ] **D** Medial sural cutaneous.
- [ ] **E** Saphenous.

1.129 Answer: D

The *sympathetic chain* gives rise to the greater, lesser and least splanchnic nerves in the thorax. These emerge from T5–L2. They are pre-ganglionic and pass through the crura of the diaphragm where they synapse on coeliac ganglia.

1.130 Answer: C

The *choroid plexus* is located in the central part and the inferior horn of the lateral ventricles.

1.131 Answer: C

The *subcostal nerve* supplies the skin of the anterior buttock between the iliac crest and the greater trochanter. The iliohypogastric nerve supplies the upper part of the buttock behind the area supplied by the subcostal nerve.

1.132 Answer: E

The *saphenous nerve* is a sensory nerve only; it supplies the skin on the medial side of the leg.

The *femoral nerve* does not travel in the adductor canal – it ends by branching superior to the adductor canal, in the femoral triangle. Knee extension would be affected in this case.

The *ilioinguinal nerve* is a branch of the lumbar plexus, which innervates muscles of the lower abdominal wall.

The *medial sural cutaneous nerve* is a branch of the tibial nerve, responsible for providing cutaneous sensation to the upper posterior calf.

The *obturator nerve* innervates the medial, adductor compartment of the thigh.

1.133 A patient presents 24 hours after a partial thyroidectomy with a hoarse voice and difficulty in breathing. Which nerve is injured?

   A Internal branch of superior laryngeal.

   B Ansa cervicalis.

   C Ansa subclavia.

   D Recurrent laryngeal.

   E External branch of superior laryngeal.

1.134 Which statement about the suprarenal glands is correct?

   A Their entire arterial supply is directly from the abdominal aorta.

   B Veins from both glands drain directly into the inferior vena cava (IVC).

   C The glands are not usually covered by renal fascia.

   D Cells that secrete adrenaline (epinephrine) and noradrenaline (norepinephrine) are innervated by pre-ganglionic fibres.

   E Fibres are from the greater thoracic splanchnic nerve.

1.133   Answer: E

The *recurrent laryngeal nerve* (RLN) runs with the inferior thyroid artery towards the lower lobes of the thyroid, and is at risk in any surgery involving the inferior thyroid artery or the inferior poles of the thyroid.

The RLN innervates all the muscles of the larynx with the exception of the cricothyroid.

The *internal branch of the superior laryngeal* runs with the superior laryngeal artery and pierces the thyrohyoid membrane.

The *ansa cervicalis* is a branch of the cervical plexus that innervates the strap muscles.

The *ansa subclavia* is part of the sympathetic trunk that loops around the subclavian artery.

The *external branch of the superior laryngeal nerve* runs with the superior thyroid artery – these are the artery and nerve that might be damaged when removing the superior lobes of the thyroid.

1.134   Answer: D

Pre-ganglionic fibres from the *greater thoracic splanchnic nerve* innervate cells that secrete catecholamines.

Pre-ganglionic sympathetic fibres from the greater thoracic splanchnic nerve directly innervate the suprarenal medulla.

The *superior suprarenal arteries* branch from the inferior phrenic artery.

The middle suprarenal artery is a direct branch of the abdominal aorta and the inferior suprarenal arteries are branches of the renal artery.

Although the vein from the right gland drains into the IVC, the vein from the left suprarenal gland drains into the left renal vein.

The suprarenal gland is covered by the renal fascia and is located in the perirenal space.

1.135 Which nerve carries post-ganglionic parasympathetic fibres to the parotid gland?

   A Auriculotemporal nerve.

   B Lesser petrosal nerve.

   C Glossopharyngeal nerve.

   D Great auricular nerve.

   E Marginal mandibular nerve.

1.136 The temporomandibular joint is characterised by all EXCEPT:

   A An articular disc.

   B Extracapsular ligaments.

   C Two joint cavities.

   D A capsule strengthened by ligaments on its lateral side only.

   E A completely flat surface for its gliding action.

1.135 Answer: A

The *auriculotemporal nerve*, a branch of the mandibular division of the trigeminal nerve (V3), carries post-ganglionic parasympathetic fibres to the parotid gland. These fibres come from the otic ganglia, where they synapse with presynaptic fibres from the glossopharyngeal nerve (CN IX).

The presynaptic fibres are carried to the otic ganglia by the *lesser petrosal nerve*, and also provide sensory innervation to the skin of anterosuperior ear, part of the external auditory meatus and the temporomandibular joint.

The *great auricular nerve* is a sensory nerve from the cervical plexus that supplies the skin of the ear and just below the ear.

The *marginal mandibular nerve* innervates the muscles of facial expression for the lower lip and chin.

1.136 Answer: E

The *temporomandibular joint* (TMJ) joint is a synovial joint with two articular cavities. Each cavity is responsible for a different movement at the joint.

The lower part of the joint is its hinge component.

When the joint moves, this hinge component initiates mandibular opening.

The upper part of the joint is the gliding component. During joint movement, this gliding cavity moves to terminate mandibular opening. The gliding cavity (not a flat surface) is the space between the articular disc and the mandibular fossa and articular eminence of the temporal bone.

There are extracapsular ligaments around the TMJ joint capsule on the lateral side only. The lateral ligament reinforces the lateral part of the capsule.

There is also an articular disc dividing the two components of the joint.

Anatomy answers

1.137 Damage of the lingual nerve before it is joined by the chorda tympani in the infratemporal fossa would cause loss of:

 A General sensation to the anterior two-thirds of the tongue.

 B General sensation to the posterior one-third of the tongue.

 C Submandibular gland secretions.

 D Taste sensation from the anterior two-thirds of the tongue.

 E Taste sensation from the posterior third of the tongue.

1.138 A child ruptured her eardrum when she inserted a pencil into her ear. The most likely nerve that may be damaged by the pencil is:

 A The auricular branch of the vagus.

 B The chorda tympani.

 C The glossopharyngeal (CN IX).

 D The lesser petrosal.

 E The auriculotemporal nerve.

1.139 Which statement is correct? The sciatic nerve can be indicated by:

 A Following the tendon of biceps femoris.

 B A point midway between the ischial tuberosity and the superior angle of the greater trochanter.

 C Nélaton's line.

 D The centre of a horizontal line from the pubic tubercle to the top of the greater trochanter.

 E A line drawn from the posterosuperior iliac spine to the posterosuperior angle of the greater trochanter.

1.137   Answer: A

The *lingual nerve* is a branch of V3, and transmits general sensation from the anterior two-thirds of the tongue. Damaging this nerve anywhere along its course would cause loss of general sensation to the anterior two-thirds of the tongue.

The *chorda tympani* carries taste fibres to the anterior two-thirds of the tongue, and presynaptic and parasympathetic fibres to the submandibular ganglion. The fibres from the chorda tympani join the lingual nerve as they travel to the submandibular ganglion and the anterior tongue.

1.138   Answer: B

The chorda tympani lies across the tympanic membrane and could therefore be damaged.

The *auricular branch* of the vagus nerve is a small branch that supplies afferent sensory innervation to the external acoustic meatus but not close to the tympanic membrane

The *glossopharyngeal nerve* and *lesser petrosal nerve* are associated with the promontory of the ear, which is on the medial wall of the middle ear.

1.139   Answer: B

The *sciatic nerve* can be indicated by a line from a point midway between the outer border of the ischial tuberosity and the posterosuperior angle of the greater trochanter to the upper angle of the popliteal fossa.

The *hip joint* may be indicated by the centre of a horizontal line from the pubic tubercle to the top of the greater trochanter.

The *common peroneal nerve* follows the line of the tendon of biceps femoris.

Nélaton's line is drawn from the anterosuperior iliac spine to the most prominent part of the ischial tuberosity. It crosses the centre of the acetabulum and the upper border of the greater trochanter.

1.140 A patient with chronic otitis media might have all the following complications EXCEPT:

A Inability to chew food.

B Loss of taste in the anterior part of the tongue.

C Mastoiditis.

D Paralysis of facial muscles.

E Deafness.

1.141 A 90-year-old man suffers a stroke resulting in right-sided paralysis. Computed tomography (CT) shows that the intracerebral haemorrhage has interrupted the blood supply to the posterior part of the frontal and the medial portions of the temporal lobes of the left cerebral hemisphere. Which vessel is affected?

A Posterior cerebral artery.

B Great cerebral vein.

C Middle cerebral artery.

D Middle meningeal artery.

E Anterior cerebral artery.

1.142 An elderly patient developed meningitis and superior sagittal sinus thrombosis a few days after sustaining a scalp laceration. Infection to the sinus initially spread through:

A Areolar tissue.

B Connective tissue.

C Epicranial aponeurosis.

D Periosteum.

E Arachnoid.

1.143 Which of the following is false with regard to the CSF?

A The CSF has its total volume replaced two to three times in 24 hours.

B The CSF passes to the third ventricle via the foramen of magendie.

C The CSF provides nutrition for glial cells.

D The CSF has a greater sodium, chloride and magnesium content than plasma.

E CSF otorrhea presents a risk of meningitis.

1.140   Answer: A

The *mandibular division of the trigeminal nerve* is not associated with the middle ear. The chorda tympani nerve travels along the lateral wall of the middle ear, running across the tympanic membrane, and could be damaged. The mastoid air cells connect to the middle ear and, therefore, an infection in the middle ear could easily spread to them.

The *facial nerve* is located on the posterior wall of the middle ear and could also be damaged by chronic infection. Chronic infection could damage the ossicles and lead to deafness.

1.141   Answer: C

The middle cerebral artery supplies:

- most of the lateral surface of the cerebral hemispheres
- the temporal pole (including the frontal, parietal, and medial portions of the temporal lobes).

The anterior cerebral artery supplies the medial and superior surfaces of the brain (including the frontal pole).

The posterior cerebral artery supplies:

- the inferior surface of the brain
- the occipital pole.

1.142   Answer: A

The areolar tissue or loose connective tissue layer of *the scalp* allows pus or blood to spread infections in this layer. This can pass into the cranial cavity through emissary veins.

1.143   Answer: B

The CSF flows from the lateral to the third ventricle via the foramen of Monro, and then into the fourth ventricle via the cerebral aqueduct. CSF rhinorrhea and otorrhea can result in meningitis as infection can spread to the meninges from the ear or nasal cavities.

1.144 **With regard to the parotid gland, which is false?**

⬜ **A** The parotid gland contains a fascial sheath, which is innervated by C2.

⬜ **B** It receives a post-ganglionic parasympathetic nerve from the otic ganglion.

⬜ **C** It contains a duct that opens into the mouth opposite the upper canine tooth.

⬜ **D** It is composed of serous acini, which contribute to the saliva.

⬜ **E** It is overlapped anteriorly by the masseter.

1.145 **Which is NOT true with regard to the pudendal nerve?**

⬜ **A** It crosses the greater sciatic foramen.

⬜ **B** It crosses the lesser sciatic foramen.

⬜ **C** It gives off the inferior haemorrhoidal nerve.

⬜ **D** It gives off the posterior cutaneous nerve of the thigh.

⬜ **E** It arises from S2–S4.

1.144   Answer: C

The *parotid gland* lies:

- anterior to the tip of the mastoid and external auditory canal
- inferior to the zygomatic arch
- superior to the lower border of the angle of the mandible.

Anteriorly, it overlaps the masseter muscle.

The parotid duct enters the oral cavity through the buccal mucosa opposite the upper second molar. It is the largest salivary gland and contains serous acini.

The secretomotor nerve arises from the parasympathetic component within the glossopharyngeal nerve. It then travels within the lesser petrosal nerve, which synapses in the otic ganglion. The post-ganglionic nerve reaches the gland via the auriculotemporal nerve.

1.145   Answer: D

The *pudendal nerve* is derived from the ventral branches of S2, S3 and S4. It passes between the piriformis and coccygeus muscles and leaves the pelvis through the greater sciatic foramen. It then crosses the spine of the ischium, and re-enters the pelvis through the lesser sciatic foramen.

It accompanies the internal pudendal vessels upwards and forwards along the lateral wall of the ischiorectal fossa, being contained in a sheath of the obturator fascia (Alcock's canal), and divides into the perineal nerve and the dorsal nerve of the penis or clitoris (its two terminal branches). Before its division it gives off the *inferior haemorrhoidal nerve*.

1.146 The artery that supplies blood to the major erectile body in both the male and female is:

- A The artery of the bulb.
- B The dorsal artery of the penis/clitoris.
- C The deep artery of the penis/clitoris.
- D The anterior labial/scrotal artery.
- E The deep external pudendal artery.

1.147 A patient presents with vertigo, ipsilateral hemi-ataxia, dysarthria and Horner's syndrome. The most likely type of stroke is:

- A Primary intracerebral haemorrhage.
- B Total anterior circulation infarct.
- C Partial anterior circulation infarct.
- D Lacunar infarct (LACI): 25%.
- E Lateral medullary syndrome/brain-stem stroke.

1.148 Which is false with regard to the facial nerve?

- A It contains only motor and sensory nerves.
- B It is important for tear production.
- C It divides into five branches after emerging from the parotid gland.
- D It is important for normal blinking reflexes.
- E It innervates the orbicularis oculi via its zygomatic and temporal branches.

1.149 Which statement about muscles acting on the shoulder is false?

- A Pectoralis major adducts the shoulder only.
- B Subscapularis medially rotates the shoulder.
- C The posterior part of deltoid extends the shoulder.
- D The central part of deltoid abducts the shoulder.
- E Extensive extension and lateral rotation of the shoulder may result in posterior dislocations.

1.146   Answer: C

The *deep artery* supplies the corpus cavernosum of the penis/clitoris. It is one of the two terminal branches of the *internal pudendal artery* – the other branch being the dorsal artery of the penis/clitoris.

The *artery of the bulb* supplies blood to the bulb of the penis and the bulb of the vestibule. It is a branch of the perineal artery.

The *superficial external pudendal artery* supplies the skin and superficial fascia of the upper medial thigh, as well as the skin of the pubic region.

1.147   Answer: E

(Posterior inferior cerebellar artery)

The *PICA syndrome* is also known as 'lateral medullary syndrome', or 'Wallenberg's syndrome', and is the most common brain-stem stroke.

It is typified by vertigo, ipsilateral hemi-ataxia, dysarthria, ptosis and miosis. Patients often have Horner's syndrome (unilateral ptosis, miosis and facial anhidrosis). PICA may arise from the vertebral artery, or as a separate branch of the basilar artery. As a result of this, most 'PICA' syndrome strokes are actually caused by vertebral artery occlusion.

1.148   Answer: C

The *facial nerve* divides into five branches within the substance of the parotid gland.

1.149   Answer: A

The clavicular head of *pectoralis major* flexes the shoulder as well. Pectoralis major also contributes to medial rotation.

1.150 Which of the following statements is NOT true?

☐ A The lacrimal gland is located behind the orbital septum.

☐ B The lacrimal gland is enclosed within a well-defined capsule.

☐ C It is a tubuloacinar structure.

☐ D It receives nerve fibres from the greater petrosal nerve.

☐ E Its lymphatic drainage is to the superficial parotid gland.

1.151 Which statement is false with regard to the temporal artery? The temporary artery:

☐ A Is a branch of the external carotid artery.

☐ B Runs on the surface of the deep fascia.

☐ C Runs under the zygomatic arch on its way to the scalp.

☐ D Is in close relation to the auriculotemporal nerve in front of the ear.

☐ E May provide significant blood supply to the intracranial circulation.

1.152 Relations of the right adrenal gland include all EXCEPT:

☐ A The IVC.

☐ B The right crus of the diaphragm.

☐ C The bare area of the liver.

☐ D The aorta.

☐ E The right kidney.

1.153 The upper end of the oesophagus is supplied mainly by:

☐ A The inferior thyroid artery.

☐ B The superior thyroid artery.

☐ C The aorta.

☐ D The transverse cervical artery.

☐ E The superior intercostal artery.

1.150   Answer: B

The lacrimal gland has no true capsule.

1.151   Answer: C

The *temporal artery* crosses the root of the zygomatic arch just in front of the auriculotemporal nerve anterior to the ear as it runs towards the scalp.

In patients with anastomosis between the internal and external carotid arteries in the forehead, the temporal artery may contribute significant blood supply to intracranial blood supply. Biopsy of this artery anterior to the ear may result in damage to the temporal branch of the facial nerve.

1.152   Answer: D

Relations of the right adrenal gland include all except the aorta.

1.153   Answer: A

The *oesophagus* is supplied by:

- Upper: the inferior thyroid artery
- Middle: by aortic branches
- Inferior: from the left gastric artery.

1.154   Which is the one true statement with regard to the hip joint?

    A   It has an articular surface of hyaline cartilage that occupies the whole of the acetabular fossa.

    B   In front, the capsule is attached just below the intertrochanteric line.

    C   The retinacular fibres bind down the nutrient arteries that pass from the trochanteric anastomosis to supply the head of the femur.

    D   The iliofemoral ligament is usually square shaped.

    E   The obturator nerve does not supply the joint.

1.155   The optic cup develops from:

    A   The prosencephalon.

    B   The telencephalon.

    C   The diencephalon.

    D   The mesencephalon.

    E   The cerebellum.

1.156   A 25-year-old woman who is 2 weeks postpartum comes to hospital with a sudden-onset headache followed by vomiting and sudden loss of consciousness. Neurological examination shows a Glasgow Coma Score (GCS) of 9/15 with bilateral papilloedema. The most probable clinical diagnosis is:

    A   Amniotic fluid embolus.

    B   Cortical vein thrombosis.

    C   Septicaemia.

    D   Pulmonary embolism.

    E   Subdural haemorrhage.

1.157   A 30-year-old man presents with sudden-onset headache. An angiogram shows a posterior communicating artery aneurysm. Which nerve is most likely to be affected?

    A   The abducens nerve.

    B   The third nerve.

    C   The optic nerve.

    D   The trigeminal nerve.

    E   The trochlear nerve.

1.154   Answer: C

The articular surface of the *hip joint* is a C-shaped concavity that does not occupy the whole of the acetabular fossa.

In front, the capsule is attached to the intertrochanteric line.

The iliofemoral ligament is the strongest and triangle shaped.

Nerve supply is from the femoral nerve, obturator nerve and nerve to quadratus femoris.

1.155   Answer: C

The *prosencephalon* consists of the diencephalon and telencephalon.

The *telencephalon* becomes the cerebrum.

The *mesencephalon* becomes the midbrain.

The *diencephalon* becomes the brain stem.

1.156   Answer: B

Cortical vein thrombosis is one of the common intracranial conditions found in the postpartum period.

1.157   Answer: B

The *third nerve* (oculomotor)) runs close to the posterior communicating artery, and so pressure from this can result in a third nerve palsy.

Anatomy answers

1.158 A 96-year-old man presents with sudden weakness of his right arm and leg followed by depressed sensorium. His wife gives a history of a fall in the bath 3 weeks ago. The most likely cause for his symptoms is:

- [ ] **A** Extradural haemorrhage.
- [ ] **B** Intraventricular haemorrhage.
- [ ] **C** Subarachnoid haemorrhage.
- [ ] **D** Intracerebral haematoma.
- [ ] **E** Subdural haemorrhage.

1.159 An 86-year-old man presents with gradual onset of ataxia, memory problems and urinary incontinence. Neurological examination reveals gait ataxia and short-term memory loss. There is no evidence of papilloedema. The most likely diagnosis is:

- [ ] **A** Normal pressure hydrocephalus.
- [ ] **B** Benign prostatic hypertrophy.
- [ ] **C** Multi-infarct dementia.
- [ ] **D** Alzheimer's disease.
- [ ] **E** Subdural haemorrhage.

1.160 Sympathetic fibres that innervate the bladder come from:

- [ ] **A** S1–S4.
- [ ] **B** L1, L2.
- [ ] **C** S4.
- [ ] **D** The inferior mesenteric ganglion.
- [ ] **E** The coeliac ganglion.

1.161 The axillary nerve crosses the humerus:

- [ ] **A** At the surgical neck of the humerus.
- [ ] **B** Opposite the midpoint of a line joining the tip of the acromion to the lower edge of the deltoid tuberosity.
- [ ] **C** About 2 cm above the centre of a line joining the tip of the acromion to the lower edge of the deltoid tuberosity.
- [ ] **D** At the lateral side of the humerus at the junction of its middle and lower thirds.
- [ ] **E** At the greater tubercle.

1.158   Answer: E

This is haemorrhage from ruptured bridging veins between the dura and the arachnoid mater. The most common presentation in the elderly is altered mental state. It may also manifest with seizures or a focal neurological deficit, headache or even falls.

1.159   Answer: A

This is the classic triad of normal pressure *hydrocephalus*.

1.160   Answer: B

Sympathetic fibres to *the bladder* come from the L1 and L2 segments of the cord via the superior and inferior hypogastric plexus.

1.161   Answer: C

The axillary nerve crosses the humerous about 2 cm above the centre of a line joining the tip of the acromion to the lower edge of the deltoid tuberosity.

1.162 Which structure is related to the right sternoclavicular joint posteriorly?

- [ ] **A** Subclavian artery.
- [ ] **B** Bifurcation of the brachiocephalic artery.
- [ ] **C** Common carotid artery.
- [ ] **D** Oesophagus.
- [ ] **E** Lymphatic duct.

1.163 The capsule of the elbow joint is weakest:

- [ ] **A** Posteriorly.
- [ ] **B** Medially.
- [ ] **C** Superiorly.
- [ ] **D** Inferiorly.
- [ ] **E** Laterally.

1.164 Which statement about the wrist is false?

- [ ] **A** The radial artery lies on the floor of the anatomical snuffbox.
- [ ] **B** The abductor pollicis longus tendon may attach to the trapezium.
- [ ] **C** Scaphoid and trapezium can be palpated in the floor of the anatomical snuff box.
- [ ] **D** Scaphoid fractures are more likely to be visible on a radiograph 10–14 days after injury.
- [ ] **E** The scaphoid may receive its blood supply through both its anterior and its posterior ends.

1.165 The following cutaneous areas and sensory roots are correctly paired EXCEPT one:

- [ ] **A** The sole of foot–S1.
- [ ] **B** The umbilicus–T10.
- [ ] **C** The groin–L1.
- [ ] **D** The little finger–T1.
- [ ] **E** The index finger–C6.

1.162   Answer: B

At the level of the right sternoclavicular joint, the brachicephalic artery divides into the right subclavian artery and right common carotid trunk.

1.163   Answer: A

The capsule of the elbow joint is weakest posteriorly.

1.164   Answer: E

The *abductor pollicis longus tendon* may indeed attach to the trapezium as well as the first metacarpal. Most of the blood supply to the scaphoid enters distally. The proximal part of the scaphoid has no blood vessels entering it and depends on vessels piercing its midportion.

1.165   Answer: D

- C5 supplies the outer aspect of the shoulder.
- C7 (the longest cervical spinous process) supplies the middle finger (the longest finger).
- C8 supplies the little finger.
- T3 lies in the axilla.
- T8, T10 and T12 supply the rib margins, umbilicus and pubis respectively.
- L3 supplies the knee.
- L5 runs diagonally from the outer aspect of the tibia to the inner aspect of the foot.
- We stand on S1 (sole of foot).
- L5 supplies the first toe and S1 the little toe.

1.166 Which statement is false with regard to the course of the subclavian artery?

☐ **A** The subclavian artery has a surface marking indicated by an arch between the sternoclavicular joint and midclavicle.

☐ **B** It passes superficially to scalenus anterior.

☐ **C** It gives off the thyrocervical trunk.

☐ **D** It arises from the brachiocephalic trunk on the right side.

☐ **E** It gives off the vertebral artery.

1.167 A long distance runner complained of swelling and pain in his shin. On physical examination, skin testing showed normal cutaneous sensation of the leg. However, muscular strength tests showed marked weakness of dorsiflexion and impaired inversion of the foot. Which nerve serves the muscles involved?

☐ **A** The common fibular nerve.

☐ **B** The deep fibular/deep perineal nerve.

☐ **C** The sciatic nerve.

☐ **D** The superficial fibular nerve.

☐ **E** The tibial nerve.

1.168 A worker falls from a height and lands on his feet. Radiographs reveal a fracture of sustentaculum tali. The muscle passing immediately beneath it that would be adversely affected is:

☐ **A** Fibularis longus.

☐ **B** Flexor digitorum longus.

☐ **C** Flexor hallucis longus.

☐ **D** Tibialis anterior.

☐ **E** Tibialis posterior.

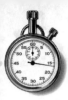

1.166   Answer: B

The surface marking of the subclavian artery is indicated by an arch between the medial end of the sternoclavicular joint and the lateral end at the midclavicle. Its course is as follows: on the right, it originates from the brachiocephalic trunk and on the left, from the arch of the aorta. It passes posterior to scalenus anterior and becomes the axillary artery at the lateral border of the first rib. Branches are vertebral, internal thoracic, deep cervical, the highest intercostal arteries and the thryocervical trunk.

1.167   Answer: B

The deep fibular nerve provides motor innervation to the anterior compartment of the leg. This compartment contains tibialis anterior, a muscle that allows for dorsiflexion and inversion of the foot. When the deep fibular nerve is affected, the only sensory loss would be on the web of skin between the first and second toes.

1.168   Answer: C

The tendon of flexor hallucius longus passes under sustentaculum tali, creating a groove in the bone. The sustentaculum tali is a shelf-like medial projection of the calcaneus, which supports the talus. If fractured, the tendon of flexor hallucis longus would be displaced from its usual position and the muscle would be affected. The fibularis longus tendon enters the foot on the lateral side. It grooves the cuboid bone and travels deep to the long plantar ligament to insert on the medial cuneiform bone. The tendon of flexor digitorum longus crosses onto the plantar surface anterior to sustentaculum tali and eventually divides into four tendons that insert into the bases of the distal phalanges of the second to fifth digits. The tendon from tibialis anterior crosses the dorsal side of the foot and inserts on the medial surface of the first cuneiform and the first metatarsal. The tibialis posterior tendon crosses under the foot on the medial side, anterior to both flexor hallucis longus and flexor digitorum longus, inserting on the navicular, the medial cuneiform and the second to fourth metatarsals.

1.169 After surgical opening of the adductor canal, a patient experienced a loss of cutaneous sensation of the medial side of the leg. Which nerve was cut?

- A The ilioinguinal nerve.
- B The femoral nerve.
- C The obturator nerve.
- D The medial sural cutaneous nerve.
- E The saphenous nerve.

1.170 With regard to the patella, which statement is false?

- A It is a sesamoid bone in the quadriceps tendon.
- B The medial border receives fibres of vastus medialis.
- C The articular surface is broader laterally.
- D The articular surface has a horizontal ridge.
- E Stellate fractures may show no displacement.

1.171 Which one statement is true with regard to approaches to the hip?

- A The anterior approach is through the interval between sartorius and gluteus medius.
- B The anterolateral approach is between tensor fascia lata and gluteus medius.
- C The posterior approach involves splitting the fibres of gluteus minimus.
- D Piriformis and obturator internus are not usually divided in the posterior approach.
- E The sciatic nerve is retracted laterally in the posterior approach.

1.172 Which statement is false with regard to the cruciate ligaments?

- A They lie within the capsule of the knee joint.
- B Lateral collateral ligament (LCL) injuries are more frequent than medial (MCL) ones.
- C The anterior cruciate attaches to the posteromedial aspect of the lateral femoral condyle.
- D The cruciate ligaments cross each other.
- E The posterior cruciate is shorter and less oblique.

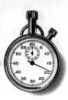

1.169 Answer: E

The saphenous nerve is a sensory nerve only; it supplies the skin on the medial side of the leg. The femoral nerve does not travel in the adductor canal – it ends by branching superior to the adductor canal, in the femoral triangle. The ilioinguinal nerve is a branch of the lumbar plexus that innervates muscles of the lower abdominal wall. The medial sural cutaneous nerve is a branch of the tibial nerve, responsible for providing cutaneous sensation to the upper posterior calf. The obturator nerve innervates the medial adductor compartment of the thigh.

1.170 Answer: D

Stellate fractures may show no displacement of fragments if the overlying quadriceps expansions and retinacula remain intact. The articular surface has a vertical ridge dividing it into a narrow medial and broader lateral surface.

1.171 Answer: B

The anterior approach is through the interval between sartorius and tensor fascia lata. The posterior approach involves splitting the fibres of gluteus maximus. Piriformis obturator internus and the gemelli are divided at their femoral attachments to expose the capsule. The sciatic nerve is retracted medially.

1.172 Answer: B

The cruciate ligaments are not within the synovial membrane but are covered on the front and sides by it.

MCL tears are more common than LCL ones but, fortunately, are more often grade I or II. They usually result from a clipping-type contact, a twist or any mechanism that forces the foot out and the knee in.

2. PHYSIOLOGY

Multiple true/false questions

2.1 **In a person with hypothermia (core temperature < 35°C):**

☐ A The O_2 dissociation curve is shifted to the left.

☐ B There may be a metabolic acidosis.

☐ C There may be U waves on the ECG.

☐ D There may be pulseless electrical activity.

☐ E Hypertension may be seen during rewarming.

2.2 **The following statements are true:**

☐ A Proprioception is carried by class Aα-fibres.

☐ B Muscle spindles are supplied by unmyelinated C-fibres.

☐ C Pain and cold sensation are carried by class Aδ-fibres.

☐ D Unmyelinated B fibres are autonomic pre-ganglionic fibres.

☐ E Class Aβ-fibres carry pressure sensation.

2.3 **With regard to carbon dioxide:**

☐ A 95% is carried in the blood as bicarbonate.

☐ B It reacts with protein amino groups to form carbaminohaemoglobin.

☐ C It dissolves in plasma more readily than oxygen.

☐ D It cannot form carbonic acid in the absence of carbonic anhydrase.

☐ E Its levels are detected by peripheral chemoreceptors.

2.4 **With regard to heart sounds:**

☐ A A third heart sound is a pathological finding.

☐ B Louder murmurs indicate more severe disease.

☐ C A fourth heart sound may be heard in heart failure.

☐ D An ejection systolic murmur may be benign.

☐ E The second heart sound correlates with mitral valve opening.

2.1   Answer: A, B, D

The O_2 dissociation curve is shifted to the left.

Hypotension may be seen as temperature increases.

J waves may be seen on the ECG.

Complications include arrhythmias, pneumonia, pancreatitis, acute renal failure and intravascular coagulation.

2.2   Answer: A, C, E

- Class Aα = motor/proprioception
- Class Aβ = touch/pressure
- Class Aδ = pain/cold
- Class Aγ = motor function to muscle spindles
- Myelinated B fibres = autonomic pre-ganglionic
- Unmyelinated C fibres = unmyelinated post-ganglionic; carry pain sensation.

2.3   Answer: B, C, E

Approximately 60% of CO_2 is carried in the blood as bicarbonate.

In plasma, CO_2 will spontaneously form carbonic acid (H_2CO_3) but the reaction is much faster when carbonic anhydrase is present.

Peripheral chemoreceptors respond to changes in P_{CO_2} and P_{O_2}.

2.4   Answer: C, D

A third heart sound is occasionally heard in young fit people. In severe stenosis reduced flow across the valve may lead to a softer murmur.

Benign ejection systolic murmurs may be heard in young patients. The second heart sound correlates with aortic valve closure.

2.5 **With regard to inotropic agents:**

☐ A Noradrenaline (norepinephrine) causes increased calcium entry into cardiac muscle cells.

☐ B Cardiac glycosides prevent sodium removal from the cell.

☐ C Acidosis is positively inotropic.

☐ D Dobutamine acts mainly at α_1-receptors.

☐ E Dopamine increases renal blood flow.

2.6 **Raised intracranial pressure (ICP) may cause the following:**

☐ A Hypotension.

☐ B Bradycardia.

☐ C Cheyne–Stokes respiration.

☐ D Neck stiffness.

☐ E Papilloedema.

2.7 **With regard to the nephron:**

☐ A Glucose is mainly reabsorbed in the proximal tubule.

☐ B The thick ascending limb of the loop of Henle actively absorbs chloride.

☐ C The distal tubule is impermeable to water in the absence of antidiuretic hormone (ADH).

☐ D The medullary collecting duct is impermeable to urea.

☐ E Calcium reabsorption in the proximal tubule is regulated by parathyroid hormone.

2.8 **Which of the following are true with regard to fluid distribution?**

☐ A Total body water is approximately 45 l in a 70-kg man.

☐ B Two-thirds of total body water is intracellular.

☐ C The majority of extracellular fluid (ECF) is in the plasma.

☐ D Lymphatic fluid in a 70-kg man is approximately 1.5 l.

☐ E Children have proportionally more total body water.

2.5   Answer: A, B, E

Acidosis is negatively inotropic because H^+ competes with Ca^{2+} for binding sites. Dobutamine acts mainly at β_1-receptors.

2.6   Answer: B, C, E

Cushing's reflex after raised ICP causes hypertension and bradycardia. Cheyne–Stokes respiration may also be seen because the midbrain is compressed. Papilloedema is a late sign, but neck stiffness is more typical of meningism.

2.7   Answer: A, B, C

Urea diffuses out of the collecting duct into the medulla before entering the ascending loop of Henle.

Parathyroid hormone regulates calcium reabsorption at the distal tubule.

2.8   Answer: A, B, D, E

The ECF is mainly interstitial fluid and is about 8.5 l in a 70-kg man. Plasma makes up about 3.5 l, lymph 1.5 l and transcellular fluid another 1.5 l.

2.9   **After major surgery the following may be seen:**

☐   **A**   A decrease in tidal volume.

☐   **B**   Atelectasis.

☐   **C**   Pneumonia.

☐   **D**   Chemical pneumonitis.

☐   **E**   Increased anatomical dead space.

2.10   **After a fracture:**

☐   **A**   Bony necrosis will occur 7 days later.

☐   **B**   A vascular pannus will form at the fracture site.

☐   **C**   Osteoblasts lay down new uncalcified bone.

☐   **D**   Granulation tissue replaces the haematoma.

☐   **E**   Lamellar bone is replaced by woven bone.

2.11   **With regard to the heart:**

☐   **A**   Vagal stimulation of the heart is absent at rest.

☐   **B**   It receives 1% of cardiac output.

☐   **C**   Myocardial blood flow occurs predominantly during diastole.

☐   **D**   The right coronary artery supplies a third of the blood flow to the left ventricle.

☐   **E**   Blood flow to the myocardium is decreased by local adenosine release.

2.12   **In spirometry:**

☐   **A**   The functional residual capacity (FRC) is the volume that remains in the lungs after complete forced expiration.

☐   **B**   The FRC may be calculated using the helium dilution technique.

☐   **C**   The vital capacity (VC) is equal to the total lung capacity (TLC) minus the inspiratory reserve volume.

☐   **D**   The FRC is decreased in elderly people.

☐   **E**   Resting tidal volume is approximately 0.5 l.

2.9   Answer: A, B, C, D

Postoperative pain results in decreased tidal volumes. Atelectasis results from increased production of viscous secretions as well as a reduced ability to cough. Aspiration of gastric contents may cause a chemical pneumonitis. Anatomical dead space is unchanged.

2.10   Answer: C, D

Bony necrosis is seen after 24–48 hours. A vascular pannus is associated with rheumatoid arthritis. A callus, however, forms at the site of a healing fracture. Osteoblasts lay down new bone. The initial callus is formed of woven bone, which is gradually replaced by stronger lamellar bone.

2.11   Answer: C, D

Tonic vagal stimulation of the heart is present even at rest, which explains why a denervated heart has a higher resting rate. The heart receives 5% of cardiac output and is mainly supplied during diastole. Local adenosine, K^+ and hypoxia result in increased blood flow to the myocardium.

2.12   Answer: B, E

The FRC is the volume that remains in the lung at the end of a normal breath. The VC is the maximum volume that an individual can expire after a single maximal inspiration. It is equal to the TLC minus the residual volume (RV) and is usually 3–6 l. The FRC is increased in elderly people because elastic tissue decreases.

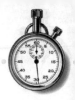

2.13   Aldosterone:

☐ **A** Is a protein hormone.

☐ **B** Is formed in the zona glomerulosa of the adrenal gland.

☐ **C** Is released in response to angiotensin II.

☐ **D** Increases sodium excretion at the nephron.

☐ **E** Binds to receptors on the cell membrane.

2.14   With regard to acid–base balance, which of the following are correct?

☐ **A** Ankylosing spondylitis may cause a respiratory acidosis.

☐ **B** Diuretics may cause a respiratory alkalosis.

☐ **C** Exercise may cause a respiratory alkalosis.

☐ **D** Vomiting may cause a metabolic acidosis.

☐ **E** Stroke may cause a respiratory acidosis.

2.15   With regard to the jugular venous pressure (JVP):

☐ **A** It reflects the intravascular volume.

☐ **B** It reflects left atrial pressure.

☐ **C** It may be raised in chronic liver disease.

☐ **D** It may be reduced in congestive cardiac failure.

☐ **E** It may be increased in pulmonary hypertension.

2.16   The thyroid hormones:

☐ **A** Decrease the activity of Na^+/K^+ ATPase.

☐ **B** Increase the rate of protein turnover.

☐ **C** Have both catabolic and anabolic actions.

☐ **D** Exert their effect over a few minutes.

☐ **E** Enhance insulin-dependent entry of glucose into cells.

2.13 Answer: B, C

Aldosterone is a mineralocorticoid. It acts at the distal convoluted tubule to reabsorb Na^+ and increase secretion of K^+ and H^+. It is a steroid hormone and hence passes through the cell membrane unhindered to act via intracellular receptors.

2.14 Answer: A, C, E

Anything causing decreased chest wall movement, such as ankylosing spondylitis or myasthenia gravis, may cause a respiratory acidosis. Diuretics increase urinary acidification and may therefore cause a metabolic alkalosis. The acid losses incurred in vomiting may cause a metabolic alkalosis. Stroke may cause a depression of the respiratory centres in the brain stem and thus cause a respiratory acidosis.

2.15 Answer: A, C, E

The JVP reflects right atrial pressure and is raised in chronic liver disease, right-sided heart failure and pulmonary hypertension.

2.16 Answer B, C, E

Thyroid hormones increase the activity of Na^+/K^+ ATPase, the rate of protein turnover, cardiac output and lipolysis. Their actions are both catabolic and anabolic but overall thyroid hormones exert an anabolic effect. Their effects take up to 4 days to reach a maximum.

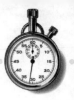

2.17   **After a meal:**

☐ **A** Cholecystokinin (CCK) is released by the gallbladder.

☐ **B** Bile salts decrease intestinal transit time.

☐ **C** Secretin stimulates acid production in the pancreatic ducts.

☐ **D** The sphincter of Oddi contracts when food is present in the duodenum.

☐ **E** Free amino acids stimulate gastrin secretion.

2.18   **Which of the following are needed to determine the cardiac output using Fick's principle?**

☐ **A** Blood from a systemic artery.

☐ **B** Blood from an antecubital vein.

☐ **C** The rate of oxygen consumption.

☐ **D** The haemoglobin concentration.

☐ **E** The heart rate.

2.19   **Cardiac output is normally related to:**

☐ **A** Body temperature.

☐ **B** Blood volume.

☐ **C** Heart rate.

☐ **D** Metabolic rate.

☐ **E** Blood pressure.

2.20   **Low blood glucose stimulates:**

☐ **A** Gluconeogenesis.

☐ **B** Glycogenolysis.

☐ **C** Gastric secretion.

☐ **D** Sweating.

☐ **E** Lipolysis.

2.17   Answer: B, E

CCK is released by duodenal cells into the bloodstream and stimulates the exocrine pancreas. Secretin stimulates the pancreatic ducts to secrete bicarbonate. The sphincter of Oddi relaxes as food arrives in the duodenum, allowing bile and pancreatic juice to enter. Peptides and free amino acids stimulate gastrin production but whole proteins do not.

2.18   Answer: A, C

Fick's principle states that the rate of diffusion is proportional to the difference in concentration. Similarly, the volume of oxygen consumed per unit time is proportional to the difference in oxygen content between arterial and venous blood. The degree of proportionality depends on the volume of blood pumped per unit time, or cardiac output (Q). Therefore, cardiac output (Q) can be calculated from the equation

Vo_2 = Cardiac output $(Ca - Cv)$

where Vo_2 is the volume of oxygen consumed per unit time, and Ca and Cv are the arterial and venous oxygen concentrations. Experimentally, the volume of oxygen consumed and the oxygen concentration in the blood can be calculated. We can then solve for cardiac output.

To use Fick's principle one must know: O_2 consumption per minute using a spirometer and a CO_2 absorber, the oxygen content of blood in the pulmonary artery and the oxygen content of blood in a peripheral artery.

2.19   Answer: all true

Cardiac output = Heart rate $\times$ Stroke volume.

2.20   Answer: all true

As well as sweating, hypoglycaemia may also cause increased appetite, headache, blurred vision and coma.

2.21 A tachycardia may be seen in:

- [ ] **A** Extracellular fluid depletion.
- [ ] **B** A Po_2 of 7 kPa.
- [ ] **C** Haemorrhage.
- [ ] **D** Raised ICP.
- [ ] **E** Vasovagal syncope.

2.22 Which of the following are essential amino acids in adults?

- [ ] **A** Histidine.
- [ ] **B** Threonine.
- [ ] **C** Glycine.
- [ ] **D** Lysine.
- [ ] **E** Methionine.

2.23 Which of the following are precursors of adrenaline (epinephrine)?

- [ ] **A** Dopamine.
- [ ] **B** Noradrenaline (norepinephrine).
- [ ] **C** Tyrosine.
- [ ] **D** Phenylalanine.
- [ ] **E** Isoprenaline.

2.24 In renal physiology:

- [ ] **A** The glomerular filtration rate (GFR) can be measured with *p*-aminohippuric acid (PAH).
- [ ] **B** The renal plasma flow is measured with inulin.
- [ ] **C** The countercurrent mechanism acts on the loop of Henle and collecting ducts.
- [ ] **D** Aldosterone acts on the distal tubules.
- [ ] **E** Of Na 99% is reabsorbed in the proximal tubules.

2.21 Answer: A, B, C

Vasovagal syncope is characterised by a bradycardia and a rapid fall in blood pressure (BP). Cushing's response seen in raised ICP involves hypertension, bradycardia and irregular respiration.

2.22 Answer: B, D, E

The eight essential amino acids in adults are phenylalanine, valine, tryptophan, threonine, isoleucine, methionone, lysine and leucine. Histidine and arginine are essential only in children.

2.23 Answer: A, B, C, D

Phenylalanine and tyrosine are the precursors in the synthesis of dopamine, which in turn is the precursor in the synthesis of adrenaline and noradrenaline.

Isoprenaline is a β-receptor agonist used in circulatory failure characterised by heart block or bradycardia.

2.24 Answer: C, D, E

The GFR is measured with inulin and, clinically, with creatinine. The renal plasma flow is measured with PAH.

2.25 **With regard to salt and water balance:**

- **A** Loss of water leads to hyperosmotic dehydration.
- **B** Loss of salt in excess of water leads to a decrease in the ECF volume.
- **C** Conn's syndrome causes hypernatraemia.
- **D** Addison's disease can cause renal loss of salt.
- **E** In the postoperative period excess intravenous dextrose causes hypertonic hyponatraemia.

2.26 **With regard to body fluids:**

- **A** Extracellular body fluid includes transcellular fluid.
- **B** Intracellular fluid can be measured with radioactive proteins.
- **C** Evans' blue is used to measure total body water.
- **D** Starling's equation governs the flow of fluid between intracellular and extracellular compartments.
- **E** Chloride is one of the major constituents of ECF.

2.27 **With regard to acid–base balance:**

- **A** Pyloric stenosis leads to hypochloraemic alkalosis.
- **B** Ureterosigmoidostomy leads to hypochloraemic acidosis.
- **C** Fistulae can cause a normal anion gap acidosis.
- **D** Artificial ventilation can cause a respiratory acidosis.
- **E** Conn's syndrome causes metabolic alkalosis.

2.28 **In respiratory physiology:**

- **A** The RV remains constant irrespective of age.
- **B** The FRC may be measured by spirometry.
- **C** The pressure–volume curve of the lung is sigmoid shaped.
- **D** The alveolar–arteriolar oxygen difference is not more than 15 mmHg.
- **E** Compared with Po_2, Pco_2 is an important marker of ventilation.

2.25 Answer: A, B, C, D

Loss of salt in excess of water leads to hyposmotic dehydration. Excess intravenous dextrose postoperatively leads to hypotonic hyponatraemia.

2.26 Answer: A, E

Plasma volume is measured with Evans' blue whereas intracellular fluid cannot be measured directly. Starling's equation governs the flow of fluid between plasma and the interstitial compartment.

2.27 Answer: A, C, E

Ureterosigmoidostomy causes hyperchloraemic acidosis. Artificial ventilation causes respiratory alkalosis by hyperventilation.

2.28 Answer: C, D, E

Residual volume increases in old age. The TLC, FRC and RV cannot be measured by spirometry. The alveolar–arteriolar difference is caused by physiological shunts in bronchioles and the coronary circulation.

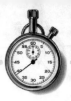

2.29 **In response to chronic hypoxia:**

▢ **A** Acute adaptation involves an increase in minute volume.

▢ **B** 2,3-DPG (2,3-diphosphoglycerate) decreases in the acute setting.

▢ **C** Erythropoietin secretion is decreased in chronic hypoxia.

▢ **D** Pulmonary hypertension does not develop in chronic adaptation.

▢ **E** Tachycardia is commonly seen during acute adaptation.

2.30 **With regard to intestinal hormones:**

▢ **A** Secretin stimulates pancreatic bicarbonate secretion.

▢ **B** Gastrin inhibits excess intrinsic factor secretion.

▢ **C** CCK stimulates gastric emptying.

▢ **D** VIP (vasoactive poplypeptide) stimulates pancreatic secretion.

▢ **E** VIP may be secreted by the large intestine.

2.31 **With regard to gastrointestinal tract (GIT) physiology:**

▢ **A** Secondary bile acids are formed in the gallbladder.

▢ **B** Enterohepatic circulation increases in ileal disease.

▢ **C** In obstructive jaundice urinary urobilinogen may be increased.

▢ **D** Brunner's glands are present in the small intestine.

▢ **E** In duodenal ulcer gastrin levels are decreased.

2.32 **With regard to fluid balance:**

▢ **A** Aqueous humor is an example of interstitial fluid.

▢ **B** Osmolality depends on the number and size of particles.

▢ **C** Children require relatively more fluid than adults.

▢ **D** Hartmann's solution is isotonic with plasma.

▢ **E** ECF loss causes change in haematocrit and plasma albumin.

2.29 Answer: A, E

Secretion of 2,3-DPG is stimulated by hypoxia, which decreases O_2 affinity for haemoglobin and thereby facilitates O_2 release. Erythropoietin production is stimulated by hypoxia, which leads to polycythaemia. Pulmonary hypertension develops during chronic adaptation.

2.30 Answer: A, D

CCK inhibits gastric emptying and stimulates pancreatic enzyme and bicarbonate secretion. Gastrin stimulates intrinsic factor secretion. VIP is secreted by the small intestine only.

2.31 Answer: D, E

The secondary bile acids are chenodeoxycholic acid and lithocholic acid. They are formed by the action of intestinal bacterial enzymes on primary bile salts in the liver. In obstructive jaundice urinary urobilinogen is decreased.

The integrity of the enterohepatic circulation is dependent on active uptake from the ileum. Bile salt malabsorption occurs in Crohns as the terminal ileum is usually affected.

2.32 Answer: C, D, E

Aqueous humor is an example of transcellular fluid. Osmolality depends on the number of particles and not on size. Change in plasma volume causes change in the haematocrit only, whereas ECF loss causes change in both the haematocrit and the albumin level.

2.33 **With regard to fluid loss:**

    A Hypovolaemia is a common cause of intraoperative metabolic acidosis.

    B Occult hypovolaemia can be detected via gut intramucosal pH.

    C A 5% glucose infusion leads to isotonic fluid expansion.

    D The CVP (central venous pressure) reflects the function of the right atrium.

    E A sustained rise in CVP of 2–4 cmH$_2$O may indicate overfilling with intravenous fluid.

2.34 **Which of the following are vasoconstrictors?**

    A Dopamine.

    B Nitric oxide.

    C Atrial natriuretic peptide (ANP).

    D Thromboxane.

    E Vasopressin.

2.35 **Causes of unilateral oedema of the limb are:**

    A Cellulitis.

    B Lymphoedema.

    C Superficial thrombophlebitis.

    D Immobility.

    E Postphlebitic limb.

2.36 **The dead space in respiratory tract ventilation:**

    A Is increased in pulmonary oedema.

    B Is decreased in pulmonary embolism (PE).

    C Includes terminal bronchioles.

    D Can be reduced by ventilation rate.

    E Is proportional to arterial oxygen concentration.

2.33   Answer: A, B

A 5% glucose infusion is an example of hypotonic fluid expansion, whereas a 0.9% saline infusion is an example of isotonic fluid expansion. The CVP reflects the function of the right ventricle. A sustained rise in CVP of 2–4 cmH_2O indicates a well-filled patient whereas a rise of more than 4 cmH_2O indicates overfilling.

2.34   Answer: A, B, D, E

Nitric oxide and adenosine are vasodilators. ANP is involved in the long term regulation of sodium and water balance, blood volume and arterial pressure. It decreases renin and aldosterone and causes systemic vasodilation.

2.35   Answer: all true

Unilateral pitting oedema	**Bilateral pitting oedema**
DVT	Cardiac failure
Superficial thrombophlebitis	Renal failure
Cellulitis	Nephrotic syndrome
Extrinsic compression of deep veins	Cirrhosis
Lymphoedema	Nutritional carcinomatosis
Immobility	

2.36   Answer: A, C

The dead space is increased in PE. It is classified as anatomical (up to the terminal bronchioles) and physiological. All areas that are perfused but not ventilated, or ventilated but not perfused, are considered dead space.

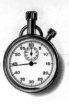

2.37 Intrinsic (intracranial) factors that regulate cerebral blood flow are:

- ☐ **A** Cardiac output.
- ☐ **B** Blood viscosity.
- ☐ **C** Cerebral vessels.
- ☐ **D** CSF pressure.
- ☐ **E** Cerebral autoregulation.

2.38 With regard to ADH:

- ☐ **A** It is released in response to an increased plasma osmolality.
- ☐ **B** Increased secretion occurs postoperatively.
- ☐ **C** It is released from the anterior pituitary gland.
- ☐ **D** It causes renal vasoconstriction.
- ☐ **E** It binds to steroid receptors.

2.39 A raised alkaline phosphatase (ALP) occurs in:

- ☐ **A** Parathyroid adenoma.
- ☐ **B** Osteomalacia.
- ☐ **C** Biliary stricture.
- ☐ **D** Bone metastases.
- ☐ **E** Recent fracture.

2.40 After trauma, a 70-kg man loses 20% of his blood volume as a result of haemorrhage. Which of the following are true?

- ☐ **A** A tachycardia will be seen.
- ☐ **B** Urine output may be normal.
- ☐ **C** Up to 750 ml of blood has been lost.
- ☐ **D** Systolic blood pressure will be normal.
- ☐ **E** Pulse pressure may be increased.

2.37   Answer: C, D, E

Cardiac output and blood viscosity are extrinsic factors that regulate cerebral blood flow.

2.38   Answer: A, B, D

ADH is released via neurosecretion from the posterior pituitary gland. It is a peptide made up of nine amino acids, formed from a larger precursor molecule produced in the hypothalamus.

2.39   Answer: all true

Hepatobiliary disease, bone disease, some malignancies and pregnancy are known to increase ALP levels. A specific assay for each isoenzyme can be used to differentiate some of these causes.

2.40   Answer: A, B, D

This represents a class II haemorrhage and the volume lost is between 750 and 1500 ml. Urine output may be low or normal. BP is usually normal, but a tachycardia will be seen. Pulse pressure is usually decreased in these patients as diastolic pressure increases.

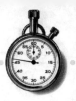

2.41 Which of the following are true with regard to absorption in the gut?

    A Vitamin B_{12} is absorbed in the terminal ileum.

    B Bile salts are absorbed throughout the ileum and proximal colon.

    C Folate is absorbed in the jejunum.

    D Magnesium is mainly absorbed in the duodenum.

    E Phosphorus is mainly absorbed in the proximal small bowel.

2.42 With regard to 5% dextrose solution:

    A It contains 278 mmol/l dextrose.

    B It provides a good source of energy in the starved patient.

    C It is hypotonic.

    D Is the fluid of choice for volume replacement in shock.

    E It is distributed throughout the total body water.

2.43 During strenuous exercise which of the following are true?

    A Systolic BP increases.

    B Pa_{CO_2} may be low.

    C Cardiac output doubles.

    D Renal blood flow is reduced.

    E Ventilatory rate increases threefold.

2.44 Which of the following are correct with regard to postoperative pyrexia?

    A On day 10 it is typically the result of the systemic response to trauma.

    B On day 5 it may be caused by a wound infection.

    C After 7–10 days it may result from a PE.

    D In the first 2 days it is typically caused by deep vein thrombosis (DVT).

    E In the first 3 days it may be the result of pulmonary atelectasis.

2.41 Answer: A, C, E

Bile salts are absorbed as part of the enterohepatic circulation in the terminal ileum. Magnesium is also mainly absorbed in the distal small intestine, whereas phosphorus is absorbed in the duodenum and proximal ileum.

2.42 Answer: A, C, E

Five per cent dextrose is isotonic when infused, but rapidly becomes hypotonic as the dextrose is metabolised. It then leaves the intravascular space and is distributed throughout the total body water. Therefore it is not ideal for shocked patients. It contains a negligible 30 kcal/l and is not therefore a good source of energy.

2.43 Answer: A, B, D

During severe exercise systolic pressure increases but diastolic pressure decreases. The cardiac output increases sixfold, the stroke volume increases twofold and the ventilatory rate increases fifteenfold. Renal blood flow is reduced.

2.44 Answer: B, C, E

Postoperative pyrexia has a number of important causes, each of which should be looked for by careful examination of the patient. The systemic response to trauma may cause a transient pyrexia, which is seen in the early postoperative period. DVT and PE are typically seen after the first week. These timescales are not absolute but are a useful rough guide.

2.45 **The rate of gastric emptying:**

☐ **A** Is enhanced by alcohol.

☐ **B** Is delayed in pregnancy.

☐ **C** Is enhanced by secretin.

☐ **D** Depends on the volume of food ingested.

☐ **E** Is enhanced by vagal stimulation.

2.46 **In pregnant women:**

☐ **A** Symptoms of hypovolaemia are seen earlier than expected.

☐ **B** Heart rate increases throughout pregnancy.

☐ **C** The GFR increases during pregnancy.

☐ **D** The minute ventilation is reduced.

☐ **E** Oxygen consumption is increased.

2.47 **Reduced urine output in severe trauma may be caused by:**

☐ **A** ADH release.

☐ **B** Haemorrhage.

☐ **C** Increased corticosteroid release.

☐ **D** Increased levels of catecholamines.

☐ **E** Decreased renin release.

2.48 **After cardiopulmonary bypass:**

☐ **A** There is a 5% incidence of stroke.

☐ **B** Acute pancreatitis may be seen.

☐ **C** Mild neurological deficits are common.

☐ **D** Most neurological deficits are reversible.

☐ **E** Thrombocytosis commonly develops.

2.49 **Glucagon:**

☐ **A** Is produced by the α cells in the pancreas.

☐ **B** Release is augmented by catecholamines.

☐ **C** Stimulates the release of insulin.

☐ **D** Is a positive inotrope.

☐ **E** Release is increased in starvation.

2.45   Answer: B, D, E

Alcohol, secretin and the presence of fat in the duodenum will all delay gastric emptying. The type and volume of food ingested determine the rate of emptying. Stimulation of the vagus nerve relaxes the pylorus.

2.46   Answer: B, C, E

As plasma volume increases during pregnancy, pregnant women can lose up to 1500 ml of their blood volume before signs of hypovolaemia are seen. Minute ventilation is increased primarily as a result of an increase in tidal volume.

2.47   Answer: A, B, C, D

Urine output is a good marker of organ perfusion.

Catecholamines, ADH and corticosteroids are all increased after trauma. In the acute setting haemorrhage should be identified and managed early.

2.48   Answer: B, C, D

Mild neurological deficits are common after cardiopulmonary bypass. They are probably a result of microemboli or hypoperfusion and are mostly reversible. The incidence of stroke is less than 1%. Pancreatitis is a risk in any open heart procedure.

2.49   Answer: all true

Glucagon is primarily released by low blood sugar directly. However, low blood sugar drives catecholamine release, which activates β-adrenoceptors on α cells, causing release of glucagon. Insulin inhibits glucagon release, but glucagon stimulates insulin release to ensure basal levels of insulin release even in hypoglycaemia.

2.50   **Glucocorticoids:**

☐ **A**   Suppress the activity of immune cells.

☐ **B**   Mimic the actions of aldosterone on the kidney.

☐ **C**   May cause stress ulceration.

☐ **D**   May cause hyperkalaemia.

☐ **E**   Are released from the kidney.

2.51   **Intracranial pressure may be reduced by:**

☐ **A**   A rise in arterial P_{CO_2}.

☐ **B**   Hyperventilation.

☐ **C**   Sitting up.

☐ **D**   Intravenous mannitol.

☐ **E**   Dexamethasone.

2.52   **The human testes secrete:**

☐ **A**   Fructose.

☐ **B**   Testosterone.

☐ **C**   FSH.

☐ **D**   Oestradiol.

☐ **E**   Progesterone.

2.53   **After removal of a kidney in a normal person:**

☐ **A**   The number of functioning nephrons is halved.

☐ **B**   The number of osmoles excreted is halved.

☐ **C**   The remaining nephrons excrete more osmotically active substances.

☐ **D**   There is increased filtration in the remaining nephrons.

☐ **E**   The ability to form dilute urine is lost.

2.50 Answer: A, B, C

Glucocorticoids are released from the adrenal glands and have a wide range of actions. High levels will suppress the immune system and can mimic mineralocorticoids causing potassium loss and sodium retention at the kidney. In prolonged stress high levels of glucocorticoids can lead to hypertension and stress ulceration.

2.51 Answer: B, C, D, E

Hyperventilation causes hypocapnia, which directly constricts the cerebral vasculature. Intravenous mannitol is an osmotic diuretic that may be used in cerebral oedema. Steroids will reduce the oedema around an intracranial lesion, allowing the pressure to be reduced.

2.52 Answer: B, D, E

The testes secrete a number of hormones including testosterone, oestradiol, inhibin, androstenedione and progesterone. Fructose is produced by the seminal vesicles and follicle-stimulating hormone (FSH) and luteinising hormone (LH) are produced by the anterior pituitary.

2.53 Answer: A, C, D

When one *kidney* is removed surgically, the number of functioning nephrons is halved.

The number of osmoles excreted is not reduced to this extent, so the remaining nephrons will be filtering and excreting more osmotically active substances.

The ability to form dilute urine is not usually lost unless there is advanced renal disease, when the osmolality of the urine becomes fixed to that of plasma.

2.54 **The GFR is affected by which of the following?**

- [ ] **A** The size of the capillary bed.
- [ ] **B** Permeability of the glomerular capillaries.
- [ ] **C** Changes in systemic blood pressure.
- [ ] **D** Efferent arteriolar constriction.
- [ ] **E** Ureteral obstruction.

2.55 **The filtration fraction:**

- [ ] **A** Is normally 16–20% of the plasma volume.
- [ ] **B** Is reduced by a slight fall in systemic blood pressure.
- [ ] **C** Is inversely proportional to renal plasma flow.
- [ ] **D** Is raised by efferent arteriolar constriction.
- [ ] **E** Is raised by afferent arteriolar constriction.

2.56 **Thyroid hormones:**

- [ ] **A** Lower circulating cholesterol levels.
- [ ] **B** Increase the rate of carbohydrate absorption from the gastrointestinal tract.
- [ ] **C** Stimulate lipolysis.
- [ ] **D** Increase the number of β-adrenergic receptors in the heart.
- [ ] **E** Stimulate oxygen consumption by the anterior pituitary.

2.57 **In the ABO system:**

- [ ] **A** A, B and O antigens are found in many tissues in addition to blood.
- [ ] **B** A and B antigens are complex oligosaccharides.
- [ ] **C** The H antigen does not persist in type O individuals.
- [ ] **D** O patients are universal recipients.
- [ ] **E** Type A individuals develop anti-B antibodies.

2.54   Answer: all of them

Glomerular filtration is affected by the same factors governing filtration across all other capillaries.

2.55   Answer: A, C, D

The *filtration fraction* is the ratio of GFR to renal plasma flow (or GFR/RPF).

A fall in systemic blood pressure causes the GFR to fall less than the RPF because of efferent arteriolar constriction, consequently causing a rise in the filtration fraction. The filtration fraction will fall if the systolic pressure falls below 70 mmHg.

2.56   Answer: A, B, C, D

Thyroid hormone stimulates O_2 consumption by metabolically active tissues, except in:

- the spleen
- the anterior pituitary
- the testes
- the lymph nodes
- the uterus
- the adult brain.

2.57   Answer: A, B, C, E

In the *ABO system*, type A and B individuals have a gene coding for a transferase that places a terminal *N*-acetylgalactosamine (group A) or galactose (group B) on the H antigen, whereas type O individuals have neither.

O patients are universal donors because they do not have either antigen.

AB patients have no circulating agglutinins and can be given any blood type.

Blood typing is performed by mixing an individual's red cells with antisera containing various agglutinins on a slide and looking for agglutination.

2.58   **Surgical removal of the lung reduces:**

☐ **A** The percentage saturation of the arterial blood with oxygen by 20%.

☐ **B** FEV$_1$ (forced expiratory volume in 1 s) by approximately 20%.

☐ **C** Exercise tolerance.

☐ **D** RV.

☐ **E** Ventilation/perfusion ratio by 50%.

2.59   **A shift of the oxygen dissociation curve to the left:**

☐ **A** Decreases the oxygen content of the blood at a given partial pressure of oxygen (Po_2).

☐ **B** Occurs in blood stored for a month.

☐ **C** Is characteristic of fetal blood.

☐ **D** Impairs oxygen delivery to the tissues at the normal tissue Po_2.

☐ **E** Occurs in cold blood.

2.60   **Ischaemic necrosis is a recognised complication of which of the following bones?**

☐ **A** Talus.

☐ **B** Pisiform.

☐ **C** Calcaneum.

☐ **D** Femoral head.

☐ **E** Scaphoid.

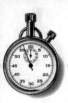

2.58   Answer: C, D

The percentage *saturation of the blood* with oxygen is not affected as a single lung can maintain oxygenation at rest.

FEV_1 is reduced by 50%.

Maximum ventilation and maximum oxygen uptake are reduced.

The residual volume is also reduced, leading to a restrictive lung disease-type picture. However, the ventilation/perfusion ratio is not affected.

2.59   Answer: B, C, D, E

The *oxygen content of the blood* is increased especially at tissue Po_2 levels.

Blood stored for several weeks does not release its oxygen content adequately.

A decreased temperature will shift the oxygen dissociation curve to the left and may reduce delivery of oxygen to tissues.

Fetal blood can take up oxygen at the lower Po_2 levels seen in the placenta, but fetal tissue Po_2 has to be low for its release to occur.

2.60   Answer: A, D, E

Fractures of the talus, scaphoid and femoral head may be complicated by *ischaemic necrosis* because of the nature of the blood supply to these bones.

Fracture lines through them result in separation of one fragment from its blood supply, in turn resulting in ischaemic necrosis.

2.61 The difference between osteoporosis and osteomalacia:

    A Is that the remaining bone in osteoporosis is normal histologically.

    B Is that major changes can be seen in the epiphyses in osteoporosis.

    C Is that pseudofractures are more common in osteomalacia.

    D Is that excess osteoid is a characteristic feature of osteomalacia.

    E Is that the total amount of bone is unchanged in osteoporosis.

2.62 The ICP will rise when:

    A Arterial P_{CO_2} falls below normal.

    B CVP rises.

    C Cerebral blood flow (CBF) increases.

    D The Valsalva manoeuvre is performed.

    E There is coughing.

2.63 Which of the following result from posterior column damage of the spinal cord?

    A Loss of pain sensation.

    B Loss of vibration sense.

    C Loss of flexor plantar response to stimulation of the sole of the foot.

    D Loss of touch sensation.

    E Loss of balance.

2.64 Loss of pancreatic juice in the duodenum may result in:

    A Undigested proteins in the stools.

    B A high prothrombin blood level.

    C Increased fat content of the faeces.

    D Higher specific gravity of the faeces.

    E All of the above.

2.61   Answer: A, C, D

Both conditions will result in reduced radiological density.

In *osteomalacia,* osteoid is laid down, which is not calcified. Epiphyseal changes are characteristic and caused by vitamin D deficiency, therefore leading to a failure of mineralisation of the osteoid. The onset occurs before they have fused. Excess osteoid formation here is characteristic. Pseudofractures are typical in this condition – a linear zone of translucency will often be seen.

In *osteoporosis* there is a reduction in bone matrix. The total amount of bone is reduced despite the cellular composition of the remaining bone being normal.

2.62   Answer: B, C, D, E

A *fall in* P_{CO_2} will cause cerebral vessels to constrict and reduce cerebral blood volume.

Increased CVP will distend intracranial veins and, hence, raise the pressure within the cranium.

The vasodilatation with increasing CBF will raise the volume of blood within the cranium.

2.63   Answer: B, D, E

The *pain fibres* travel in the spinothalamic tracts.

The *flexor plantar reflex* is not a component of the posterior column fibres.

2.64   Answer: A, C, D

Without pancreatic juice, there will be a lack of trypsin and chemotrypsin as well as a lack of lipase, resulting in a higher fat and protein content of the stools with a tendency for the faeces to putrefy. The faecal matter will have a lower specific gravity and stools may float in the pan.

Vitamin K is a fat-soluble vitamin and, therefore, there will be a reduced prothrombin level in the blood.

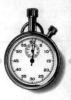

2.65 **Secretion of gastric juice:**

☐ A Is increased by food stimulating mucosal cells of the pyloric region.

☐ B Is associated with a fall in blood pH as bicarbonate enters the circulation.

☐ C Is stimulated by vagal nerve fibres.

☐ D Is essential for absorption of folate.

☐ E Is essential for absorption of vitamin B_{12}.

2.66 **Stimuli decreasing growth hormone secretion include which of the following?**

☐ A REM (rapid eye movement) sleep.

☐ B Glucose.

☐ C Cortisol.

☐ D Free fatty acids.

☐ E Fasting.

2.65 Answer: A, C, E

The three phases of gastric regulation:

a. cephalic phase
   i. initiated by parasympathetic activation (vagal innervation)
   ii. cortical (smell, thoughts, etc.) activation of medulla
   iii. medulla activates gastric juice secretion
   iv. medulla activates gastrin secretion
   v. medulla activates smooth muscle 'churning'
b. gastric phase
   i. food mass and chemicals trigger parasympathetic reflex
   ii. enhance parasympathetic activation of stomach
   iii. activate and enhance emptying of chyme into duodenum
c. intestinal phase
   i. chyme enters duodenum
   ii. three hormones secreted from small intestine mucosa:

     gastric inhibitory peptide (GIP)
     secretin
     cholecystokinin (CCK)

Absorption sites:

Iron = duodenum
Folate = jejunum (intestinal conjugase)
B12 = ileum

Folate absorption decreased with oral contraceptives, alcohol, phenytoin, pure vegan diet

B12 absorption decreased with bacterial overgrowth, pernicious anemia, Crohn's disease

2.66 Answer: A, E

Factors increasing *growth hormone* secretion include:

- exercise
- fasting
- stress
- a protein meal
- hypoglycaemia
- REM sleep.

2.67 **With regard to functional residual capacity (FRC):**

    A It can be increased by using continuous positive airway pressure (CPAP).

    B It is reduced by pregnancy.

    C It is increased by general anaesthesia.

    D It can be measured by spirometry.

    E It is the volume of air remaining in the lungs at the end of a tidal breath.

2.68 **With regard to the dead space:**

    A Alveolar dead space added to anatomical dead space forms the physiological dead space.

    B The anatomical component is approximately 150 ml.

    C Physiological dead space is increased by positive pressure ventilation.

    D Physiological dead space is increased by pulmonary emboli.

    E Increases in dead space raise the Pa_{CO_2}.

2.69 **In control of respiration:**

    A Central chemoreceptors are responsible for 50% of the response to Pa_{CO_2}.

    B Central chemoreceptors are sensitive to H^+ concentration.

    C Peripheral chemoreceptors are slower to respond to Pa_{CO_2}.

    D Anaemia has an effect on the peripheral chemoreceptors only.

    E Peripheral chemoreceptors respond to fever.

2.70 **With regard to pulse oximetry:**

    A It is affected by coloured nail varnish.

    B Carboxyhaemoglobin causes an under-estimation of saturation.

    C It is affected by methylene blue.

    D It monitors heart rate.

    E It does not quantify the ability to eliminate carbon dioxide.

2.67   Answer: A, B, E

FRC is reduced by:

- pregnancy
- general anaesthesia
- lung disease.

Supine positioning is measured by helium dilution.

2.68   Answer: all true

2.69   Answer: B, E

Central chemoreceptors are responsible for 80% of the response.

Peripheral chemoreceptors: oxygen tension ($Paco_2$) changes, rather than changes in content, generate impulses.

2.70   Answer: A, C, D, E

Carboxyhaemoglobin causes an over-estimation of saturation.

2.71 **In the central venous pressure waveform:**

   A The x descent corresponds with atrial relaxation.

   B The c wave refers to atrial relaxation.

   C The y descent is the atria emptying as blood enters the ventricle.

   D It fluctuates with respiration.

   E The a wave is ventricular contraction.

2.72 **On the intensive care (ICU):**

   A Level 3 care implies a nurse:patient ratio of 1:1.

   B Nurse staffing should be based on patient dependency rather than bed numbers.

   C Costs for those requiring level 3 care are three times those of a ward patient.

   D Level 1 patients can be cared for on an acute ward with support from a critical care team.

   E Mechanical ventilation in a patient (who is expected shortly to die) for the purposes of organ donation.

2.73 **In innervation of the lower urinary tract:**

   A The cerebral cortex is important in having an overall inhibitory control over the detrusor muscle.

   B The detrusor muscle is supplied by both parasympathetic and sympathetic nerves.

   C The levator ani is supplied by the hypogastric nerves

   D Destruction of the pons causes voiding difficulties.

   E Lesions below the level of the pons result in detrusor hyperreflexia.

2.74 **With regard to intracranial pressure:**

   A When raised above 25 mmHg, it may result in brain herniation.

   B When raised above 25 mmHg, it may result in a reduced cerebral perfusion pressure.

   C It can be monitored using a subdural catheter.

   D The normal range is 0–10 mmHg.

   E It is normal after a stroke.

2.71 Answer: A, C, D

The *c wave* refers to the rise in atrial pressure produced by bulging of the tricuspid valve into the atria during isovolumetric ventricular contraction.

The *a wave* is atrial contraction.

2.72 Answer: A, B, C, D

Closed units have better patient outcomes than open ones. Responsibility for the patient lies with the admitting consultant in an open unit and with the intensive care consultant in a closed one.

2.73 Answer: A, B, D, E

The levator ani is somatic via the pudendal nerves S2–4.

2.74 Answer: A, B, C, D

Elevation of intracranial pressure after a *stroke* causes impaired blood flow to the brain as a result of a fall in cerebral perfusion pressure.

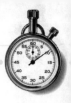

2.75 Outcome of traumatic brain injury is worse in patients with:

- A Hyperpyrexia.
- B Hypoxia.
- C Hyperglycaemia.
- D A cerebral perfusion pressure below 70, which is associated with a worse prognosis.
- E Reduced intracranial pressure.

2.76 The following are true with regard to brain-stem death reflex testing:

- A All of them involve cranial nerves.
- B All of them are consensual reflexes.
- C The only nerves tested are II, III, IV and IX.
- D During cold caloric testing nystagmus is towards the side tested.
- E Before testing the cranial nerves, the core temperature should be more than 35°C.

2.77 With regard to anticonvulsants:

- A Phenytoin should be avoided in pregnant women.
- B Carbamazepine can cause agranulocytosis.
- C Clonazepam is the drug of choice in myoclonic seizures.
- D Gabapentin has few drug interactions.
- E Phenobarbital is used in status epilepticus.

2.78 In cerebral abscesses:

- A Up to 25% have no detectable source.
- B Pulmonary abnormalities are a risk factor.
- C Differential diagnosis includes metastases.
- D Sinus thrombosis is a complication.
- E Lumbar puncture should be done in all cases.

2.75 Answer: A, B, C, D

Outcome of *traumatic brain injury* is worse in patients with raised intracranial pressure.

2.76 Answer: A, B, E

During *brain-stem death reflex* testing, the nerves tested are VIII, IX and X, and nystagmus is towards the opposite side.

2.77 Answer: A, B, C, D

Lorazepam/diazepam is usually the *first-line treatment*.

2.78 Answer: A, B, C, D

In cerebral absecesses:

up to 25% have no detectable source;

pulmonry abnormalities are a risk factor;

differential diagnosis includes metastases;

sinus thrombosis is a complication.

2.79   **With regard to hydrocephalus:**

  - **A**   Aqueductal stenosis causes a communicating hydrocephalus.
  - **B**   Hydrocephalus in the Arnold–Chiari malformation is always the result of cerebellar tonsillar herniation.
  - **C**   Ventriculoperitoneal shunting is the first-line treatment.
  - **D**   It can occur in subarachnoid haemorrhage.
  - **E**   It can be associated with craniofacial anomalies.

2.80   **With regard to Cushing's syndrome:**

  - **A**   It can be caused by lung tumours.
  - **B**   ACTH levels are elevated in hypothalamic tumours.
  - **C**   Nelson's syndrome is caused by ACTH.
  - **D**   Cushing's disease is the result of excessive ACTH.
  - **E**   The dexamethasone suppression test helps to distinguish patients with excess production of ACTH as a result of pituitary adenomas from those with ectopic ACTH-producing tumours.

2.81   **With regard to cerebral metastases:**

  - **A**   50% of cerebral metastases are solitary.
  - **B**   Most cerebral metastases are located in the cerebellum.
  - **C**   The lungs are the most common source.
  - **D**   Patients clinically present with headache and vomiting.
  - **E**   Whole brain radiotherapy (WBRT) should be given in all cases.

2.82   **In the management of carotid disease:**

  - **A**   Aspirin is proven to reduce vascular events.
  - **B**   There is inconclusive evidence to support the role of dypyridamole when compared with aspirin alone.
  - **C**   Lipid-lowering drugs have a role in reducing the risk of a cerebrovascular accident (CVA).
  - **D**   Carotid endarterectomy has a higher risk in females.
  - **E**   Carotid endarterectomy should not be considered in patients who are asymptomatic.

2.79   Answer: C, D, E

Aqueductal stenosis results in non-communicative or obstructive hydrocephalus and can also cause the Arnold–Chiari malformation.

Hydrocephalus can be treated with ventriculoperitoneal shunting but ventriculostomy is also used.

2.80   Answer: A, B, E

Nelson's syndrome is caused by melanin-stimulating hormone.

Cushing's disease is from the pituitary, and the cells in a pituitary adenoma causing Cushing's disease are typically basophilic.

2.81   Answer: A, C, D

Most *cerebral metastases* are located in the cerebral hemispheres.

Melanoma and large cell lung cancer are radioresistant.

2.82   Answer: A, B, C, D

In the management of cartoid disease:

aspirin is proven to reduce vascular events;

there is inconclusive evidence to support the role of dypyridamole when compared with aspirin alone;

lipid-lowering drugs have a role in reducing the risk of a cerebrovascular accident (CVA);

cartoid endarterectomy has a higher risk in females.

2.83 **Low-molecular-weight heparins:**

☐ **A** Have molecular masses between 2000 and 8000 Da.

☐ **B** Act by inhibiting factor V and binding to anti-thrombin III.

☐ **C** Reduce the risk of deep vein thrombosis (DVT) by 70%.

☐ **D** Are more expensive than conventional heparin.

☐ **E** Act by reducing the proportion of factors VII, IX and X.

2.84 **Stones in the salivary glands:**

☐ **A** Lead to pain and swelling worse at mealtimes.

☐ **B** Are most commonly seen in middle-aged men.

☐ **C** In 80% of cases affect the parotid gland.

☐ **D** Have a higher proportion of submandibular stones that are radio-opaque than the parotid.

☐ **E** Usually have an infectious aetiology.

2.85 **Causes of hypercalcaemia include:**

☐ **A** Addison's disease.

☐ **B** Immobility.

☐ **C** Chronic renal failure.

☐ **D** Thiazide diuretics.

☐ **E** Familial hypocalciuric hypercalcaemia.

2.86 **Which of the following cause hyperchloraemic acidosis?**

☐ **A** Duodenal fistula.

☐ **B** Ileostomy.

☐ **C** Ileo-ureteric implant.

☐ **D** Pyloric stenosis.

☐ **E** Renal tubular acidosis (RTA).

2.83 Answer: A, C, D

Low-molecular-weight *heparin* (LMWH) acts by inhibiting factor V and binding to factor X.

2.84 Answer: A, B, C

Stones in the salivary glands lead to pain and swelling worse at mealtimes, are most commonly seen in middle-aged men. In 80% of cases, stones in the salivary glands affect the parotid gland.

2.85 Answer: A, B, D, E

Chronic renal failure usually causes hypocalcaemia.

2.86 Answer: A, B, C, E

Pyloric stenosis would result in a hypochloraemic alkalosis. In RTA there is usually reduced urinary excretion of K+ coupled with a movement of K+ out of cells into the extracellular fluid. Type 1 RTA is more common and caused by a distal tubular defect that is abnormally permeable to H+ so it diffuses back into the plasma. In type 2 RTA, bicarbonate reabsorption in the proximal collecting tubule is impaired.

2.87 Which is true with regard to a cancer of the anal canal?

    A It arises above the dentate line.

    B Radiotherapy has replaced radical surgery for most anal cancers.

    C It is unlikely to be treatable with radiotherapy.

    D Examination under anaesthetic is not necessary.

    E Local resection would be indicated for a 4 cm diameter tumour.

2.88 Which of the following are stimuli for release of cortisol?

    A Stress.

    B Exercise.

    C Fever.

    D Hypoglycaemia.

    E Hyperkalaemia.

2.89 The static recoil pressure of the lung (alveolar pressure minus intrapleural pressure):

    A Is decreased in the lungs without surfactant.

    B Decreases near total lung capacity (TLC).

    C Increases when lung volume increases.

    D Can be measured only in excised lungs.

    E Decreases when lung volume increases.

2.90 Which statement is incorrect? The renal clearance for:

    A Inulin is about 125 ml/min in a normal young adult.

    B Phosphate increases when parathyroid hormone (PTH) secretion is stimulated.

    C Glucose is normally zero.

    D Free water decreases when ADH (antidiuretic hormone) secretion increases.

    E A substance that is filtered and reabsorbed is higher than the clearance of inulin.

2.87   Answer: A, B, D

Cancer of the anal canal spreads to superior haemorrhoidal nodes.

Radiotherapy has replaced radical surgery for most anal cancers, and is more likely to be treatable in this way compared with cancer below the dentate line.

Local resection is indicated in tumours of the anal margin with diameter of < 2 cm and no invasion of the sphincters on magnetic resonance imaging.

2.88   Answer: A, B, C, D

Stress, exercise, fever and hypoglcaemia are stimuli for release of cortisol.

2.89   Answer: A, B, C, D

Measured under static conditions, the *alveolar pressure* will be the same as the body surface (0) and the pleural pressure will be negative (–) relative to the body surface.

Pleural pressure becomes more negative as lung volume is increased by inspiration.

Thus, the recoil pressure of the lung (alveolar–pleural; zero minus a negative = a positive value) becomes more positive or increases.

2.90   Answer: A, C, D

The *clearance of inulin* is equal to the glomerular filtration rate (GFR).

PTH (parathyroid hormone) decreases phosphate reabsorption from the proximal tubule and the rate of excretion increases.

Normally, all of the glucose that is filtered at the glomerulus is reabsorbed in the proximal tubule. No glucose is excreted in the urine.

ADH decreases water excretion, causing the urine to become more concentrated so that the free water clearance decreases and becomes negative.

A substance that is reabsorbed by the renal tubules will have a lower clearance than that of inulin, which is only filtered.

2.91 **With regard to the body fluids:**

A In a 70-kg man the total body water (TBW) in litres represents approximately 60% of the body weight.

B Two-thirds of the TBW is located in the extracellular fluid (ECF) and one-third in the intracellular fluid (ICF).

C The normal range for the plasma Na^+ concentration is 135–145 mmol/l.

D The major ion determining the osmolarity of the ECF (extracellular fluid) is Na^+.

E Most of the calcium ions in the body fluids are intracellular.

2.92 **Proximal tubule reabsorption of bicarbonate:**

A Is mostly in exchange for Na^+.

B Is inhibited by decreases in cell pH.

C Is stimulated by high levels of angiotensin II.

D Is much more than absorption in the collecting ducts.

E Is inhibited by acetazolamide.

2.93 **With regard to transmission of pain:**

A Aδ-fibres are susceptible to local anaesthetics.

B C-fibres are susceptible to local anaesthetics.

C C-fibres may be sensitised.

D C-fibres are responsible for dull and prolonged pain.

E C-fibres are responsible for early sharp pain.

2.91 Answer: A, C, D

TBW is about 42 l in a 70-kg man.

Two-thirds (28 l) are located in the ICF and a third (14 l) in the ECF.

The *normal plasma osmolarity* is about 290 mosmol/l – 280 mosmol being contributed by sodium chloride and sodium bicarbonate.

The Ca^{2+} concentration in the ICF is very low.

2.92 Answer: A, C, D, E

Proximal reabsorption HCO_3^- is stimulated by decreases in cell pH. This acutely activates Na^+/H^+ exchange and chronically induces expression of the co-transporters.

High levels of *angiotensin II* also stimulate Na^+/H^+ exchange.

The amount of HCO_3^- reabsorbed is much smaller in the collecting ducts than in the proximal tubule.

Acetazolamide interferes with proximal reabsorption of $NaHCO_3$, and induces an osmotic diuresis.

2.93 Answer: B, C, D

Aδ-fibres: myelinated, large fibres (and similar to C-fibres may be sensitised). They are resistant to local anaesthetics but susceptible to pressure, inactivated with higher temperature and responsible for the early and initial brief sharp pain.

C-fibres: non-myelinated, small and respond to any noxious stimuli. Susceptible to local anaesthetics and responsible for the dull prolonged pain.

2.94   **Fresh frozen plasma (FFP):**

☐ **A** Contains all clotting factors.

☐ **B** Should be used immediately after thawing.

☐ **C** That is ABO compatible should be used.

☐ **D** Is produced from plasma.

☐ **E** Has a usual starting dose for a 70-kg person of 50 ml/kg.

2.95   **Bone formation is enhanced by:**

☐ **A** Insulin.

☐ **B** Glucocorticoids.

☐ **C** Growth hormone.

☐ **D** Parathyroid hormone.

☐ **E** Thyroid hormone.

2.94   Answer: A, B, C, D

FFP is produced from plasma from a single donation.

Each 150 ml bag contains:

- all clotting factors
- albumin
- γ-globulin.

FFP must be used immediately after thawing and must be ABO compatible. It is plasma frozen to –20°C.

The usual starting dose is 10–15 ml/kg (equivalent to four packs of FFP for a 70-kg person), which raises the coagulation levels 12–15%.

Premenopausal women who are Rh-D negative must receive Rh-D-negative FFP.

2.95   Answer: A, C, E

Glucocorticoids:

- They lower serum Ca^{2+} levels by inhibiting osteoclast formation and activity.
- Over long periods, they cause osteoporosis by decreasing bone formation and increasing bone resorption.
- They decrease the absorption of Ca^{2+} from the intestine by an anti-vitamin D action and increase its renal excretion. Therefore, the decrease in serum Ca^{2+} concentration increases the secretion of PTH, and bone resorption is facilitated.

Growth hormone: increases Ca^{2+} excretion in the urine, but it also increases intestinal absorption of Ca^{2+}, and this effect may be greater than the effect on excretion, with a resultant positive Ca^{2+} balance.

Thyroid hormones: cause hypercalcaemia, hypercalciuria and osteoporosis.

Oestrogen: prevents osteoporosis, probably by a direct effect on osteoblasts.

Insulin: increases bone formation, and there is significant bone loss in untreated diabetes.

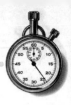

2.96 **With regard to the chemoreceptor trigger zone (CTZ):**

- [ ] **A** It is a group of cells situated close to the area postrema on the floor of the fourth ventricle.
- [ ] **B** It is situated outside the blood–brain barrier.
- [ ] **C** Ondansetron is an antagonist of receptors in this area.
- [ ] **D** It is also linked with the control of blood pressure, food intake and sleep.
- [ ] **E** Metoclopramide does not have an effect here.

2.97 **Factors that can alter the amount of K$^+$ secreted in the distal tubules include:**

- [ ] **A** The rate of flow of fluid in the tubules.
- [ ] **B** Na$^+$ reabsorption.
- [ ] **C** Acidosis.
- [ ] **D** Aldosterone.
- [ ] **E** High K$^+$ levels.

2.96   Answer: A, B, C, D

The *CTZ* is a group of cells situated close to the area postrema on the floor of the fourth ventricle. This area is extremely vascular and situated outside the blood–brain barrier, making it vulnerable to circulating drugs and toxins. It is thought to have a major impact on the activity of the vomiting centre.

The CTZ is also sensitive to systemic stimuli and linked with the control of blood pressure, food intake and sleep.

Two important *neurotransmitters* located here are:

- dopamine
- 5-hydroxytryptamine (5-HT, serotonin).

Antagonists of these will have an indirect effect on the vomiting centre to reduce nausea and vomiting.

In addition to having an effect on the CTZ, *metoclopramide* has prokinetic actions on the gut, promoting gastric emptying, and increases the barrier pressure of the lower oesophageal sphincter.

2.97   Answer: all true

K^+ secretion is proportional to the rate of flow.

Increasing the flow limits the build-up of K^+ in the tubule, which would otherwise increase and inhibit further secretion.

K^+ secretion is dependent on Na^+ reabsorption. The greater the amount of Na^+ reabsorbed, the more K^+ is secreted. This means that K^+ secretion will increase when there is decreased Na^+ in the distal tubular fluid.

K^+ secretion will increase when Na^+ absorption is increased, which is under the control of aldosterone and the atrial natriuretic peptide (ANP) and, hence, also dependent on intravascular volume and blood pressure.

High K^+ levels stimulate aldosterone secretion and act as negative feedback to maintain levels.

Na^+ is also reabsorbed in exchange for H^+. K^+ secretion is decreased when there is increased H^+ secretion, eg when a patient is acidotic.

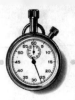

2.98   **Glucagon secretion is stimulated by:**

- [ ] **A**   Amino acids.
- [ ] **B**   Exercise.
- [ ] **C**   Gastrin.
- [ ] **D**   Secretin.
- [ ] **E**   Hyperglycaemia.

2.99   **Factors affecting end-diastolic volume include:**

- [ ] **A**   Ventricular wall stiffness.
- [ ] **B**   Blood volume.
- [ ] **C**   Intrapericardial pressure.
- [ ] **D**   Intrathoracic pressure.
- [ ] **E**   Standing.

2.100   **With regard to venous pressure in the head:**

- [ ] **A**   In the upright position the neck veins collapse above a point where the venous pressure is zero.
- [ ] **B**   The dural sinuses cannot collapse.
- [ ] **C**   The pressure in collapsed segments of vein is subatmospheric.
- [ ] **D**   The pressure in the dural sinuses is subatmospheric.
- [ ] **E**   A, B and C are correct.

2.98 Answer: A, B, C, D

Secretion of *glucagon* is stimulated by:

- hypoglycaemia
- amino acids
- CCK
- gastrin
- exercise
- infections
- β-adrenergic stimulators
- cortisol.

It is inhibited by:

- insulin
- free fatty acids
- ketones
- α-adrenergic stimulators
- secretin
- somatostatin.

2.99 Answer: A, B, C, D

Standing decreases venous return and, therefore, cardiac filling in diastole.

An increase in the normal negative *intrathoracic pressure* increases the pressure gradient along which blood flows to the heart.

An increase in intrapericardial pressure limits the extent to which the ventricles can fill.

2.100 Answer: A, B, D

In the upright position, the *neck veins* collapse above a point where the venous pressure is zero and the pressure all along the collapsed segments is close to zero. The *dural venous sinuses* have rigid walls and cannot collapse. The pressure in them in the sitting or standing position is, therefore, subatmospheric.

2.101 Which of the following does not penetrate the blood–brain barrier?

☐ **A** Water.

☐ **B** Carbon dioxide.

☐ **C** Steroid hormones.

☐ **D** Polypeptides.

☐ **E** Glucose.

2.102 Which statements are false? When blood flows from the venules to the large veins:

☐ **A** Its average velocity increases.

☐ **B** The pressure falls.

☐ **C** The total cross-sectional area of the vessels increases.

☐ **D** The velocity decreases.

☐ **E** The total cross-sectional area of the vessels decreases.

2.101 Answer: A, B, C, E

Water, CO_2, O_2 and the lipid-soluble free forms of steroid hormones penetrate the brain easily.

H^+ and HCO_3^- have a slower penetration.

Proteins and polypeptides do not penetrate the *blood–brain barrier*.

2.102 Answer: C, D

When *blood flows from the venules to the large veins* its average velocity increases as the cross-sectional area of the vessels decreases.

In the great veins, the velocity of the blood is a quarter that of the aorta, averaging 10 cm/s, but it is posture dependent.

Single best answer questions

2.103 **Which one of the following is false with respect to the thyroid gland**

☐ **A** It enlarges during pregnancy.

☐ **B** It actively absorbs iodine.

☐ **C** The posterior pituitary secretes thyroid-stimulating hormone (TSH).

☐ **D** T_3 (triiodothyronine) is more physiologically active than T_4 (thyroxine).

☐ **E** Thyroid hormones increase expression of Na^+/K^+ ATPase.

2.104 **Which of the following is true with respect to baroreceptors?**

☐ **A** The aortic arch baroreceptors are more sensitive than the carotid receptors.

☐ **B** An increase in arterial pressure decreases baroreceptor firing.

☐ **C** Aortic baroreceptors are innervated by the sinus nerve.

☐ **D** Central connections are to the medulla oblongata.

☐ **E** Low-pressure baroreceptors are found in the cardiac ventricular walls.

2.105 **With regard to saliva, which of the following is untrue?**

☐ **A** The parotid gland secretes mainly serous saliva.

☐ **B** Approximately 500 ml is produced daily.

☐ **C** It contains more sodium than plasma.

☐ **D** It is composed of 65% water.

☐ **E** It is of a higher osmolality in a resting gland than in a stimulated gland.

2.106 **Which of the statements is correct?**

☐ **A** In the cardiac cycle the rate of ejection of stroke volume is uniform throughout the ejection period.

☐ **B** Positive end-expiratory pressure (PEEP) ventilation decreases CVP.

☐ **C** Fick's method is used to calculate cardiac index.

☐ **D** The thermodilution principle uses warm saline to measure cardiac output.

☐ **E** Tachycardia causes an increase in diastolic BP.

2.103   Answer: C

The anterior pituitary secretes TSH.

2.104   Answer: D

Carotid baroreceptors are more sensitive than aortic baroreceptors. The carotid receptors are innervated by the sinus nerve, a branch of cranial nerve IX, whereas the aortic receptors are innervated by cranial nerve X. The rate of firing increases with increased blood pressure. The low pressure cardiopulmonary receptors are located within the atrial walls and great veins.

2.105   Answer: A

The parotid gland produces watery, proteinaceous saliva (secreted by the serous cells of the gland). The sublingual gland secretes mucinous saliva and the submandibular glands produce a mixed serous and mucinous saliva. Saliva contains more potassium and less sodium than plasma and is 99% water. Salivary osmolality increases as the secretion rate increases, reaching about 70% of plasma osmolality at maximal secretion rates. The pH changes from being slightly acidic (at rest) to basic (pH 8) at ultimate stimulation. This increase in alkalinity is due to the increase in HCO_3^- in the saliva. At low flow rates of saliva secretion, Na^+ is actively absorbed, Cl^- passively absorbed, but K^+ and HCO_3^- are secreted as the saliva moves out of the ducts into the mouth. However, at higher flow rates, salivary ducts are not as efficient in reabsorbing Na^+ and Cl^- because their levels now more closely approach those of the plasma. Amylase and mucus also increase in concentration after stimulation.

2.106   Answer: E

The ejection of stroke volume in the first third of systole is 70% (rapid ejection phase). PEEP ventilation increases CVP. Fick's method is used to calculate cardiac output. The thermodilution principle uses cold saline to measure cardiac output.

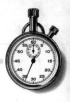

2.107 Which statement is NOT true with regard to brown fat?

A   Brown fat is more abundant in children than in adults.

B   It is richer in mitochondria than normal fat.

C   It is more vascular than normal fat.

D   It can generate more heat when parasympathetic nerves are stimulated.

E   It is more important in infants than shivering.

2.108 Which of the following will cause the greatest increase in urinary potassium excretion?

☐ **A**   Calcium chloride.

☐ **B**   Mannitol.

☐ **C**   Spironolactone.

☐ **D**   Ethanol.

☐ **E**   Furosemide.

2.109 Which one of the following statements regarding withdrawal reflexes is false?

☐ **A**   Initiated by nociceptive stimuli.

☐ **B**   Prepotent.

☐ **C**   Prolonged if the stimulus is strong.

☐ **D**   Affected by transsection of the spinal cord.

☐ **E**   Dependent on local sign for their exact pattern.

2.110 Which of the following does NOT have an analgesic effect?

☐ **A**   Substance P antagonists.

☐ **B**   Midazolam.

☐ **C**   Adrenergic antagonists.

☐ **D**   Morphine.

☐ **E**   Anandamide.

2.107   Answer: D

Metabolic activity in *brown fat* is stimulated by sympathetic activity.

It is richer in mitochondria, has a higher metabolic rate and is, therefore, more vascular than normal fat. Infants do not shiver well.

2.108   Answer: E

Loop diuretics such as furosemide inhibit the $Na^+/K^+/2Cl^-$ co-transporters in the thick segment of the loop of Henle.

Thiazides act by inhibiting Na^+/Cl^- co-transport in the distal tubule.

Both increase the delivery of sodium to the Na^+/K^+ exchange area in the collecting ducts, facilitating K^+ excretion.

2.109   Answer: D

Withdrawal reflexes are prepotent (i.e. they pre-empt any other reflex activity taking place in the spinal pathways).

Stronger stimuli do cause a more prolonged response.

The response depends on the location of the stimulus, because it serves to remove the limb from the irritating stimulus (called *local sign*).

2.110   Answer: B

Midazolam is a potent amnesic and hypnotic that produces a greater decrease in BP in hypovolaemia than diazepam.

Despite the relatively short half-life of midazolam, extensive distribution can cause prolonged sedation.

Anandamide, the ethanolamide of arachidonic acid, is an endogenous cannabinoid. It is analgesic in inflammatory and neuropathic pain.

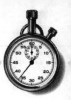

2.111 Secretion of which of the following organs does NOT primarily occur at night?

- [ ] **A** Insulin.
- [ ] **B** ACTH.
- [ ] **C** Growth hormone.
- [ ] **D** Melatonin.
- [ ] **E** Prolactin.

2.112 Left ventricular failure (LVF) does NOT cause which of the following?

- [ ] **A** An increased left atrial pressure.
- [ ] **B** A raised left ventricular end-diastolic volume (LVEDV).
- [ ] **C** Reduced lung compliance.
- [ ] **D** Increased pulmonary capillary pressure.
- [ ] **E** Pulmonary oedema on standing.

2.113 Which statement is true? In hypoxia:

- [ ] **A** Exercising muscle decreases the rate of lactate formation.
- [ ] **B** Exercising muscle results in a respiratory acidosis at high altitude.
- [ ] **C** In smokers the condition results partly from the carbon monoxide content of the blood.
- [ ] **D** The condition is alleviated by treatment with beta receptor antagonists.
- [ ] **E** The cardiac failure is of the hypoxic type.

2.114 Severe pain will NOT result in which of the following?

- [ ] **A** Fall in blood pressure as a result of a fall in vascular resistance in muscle.
- [ ] **B** Fall in heart rate.
- [ ] **C** Vomiting.
- [ ] **D** Suppression of cortisol secretion.
- [ ] **E** Sweating.

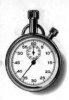

2.111   Answer: A

Secretion of insulin does not primarily occur at night.

2.112   Answer: E

In LVF:

- The left atrial pressure rises because there is inadequate emptying of the left ventricle in systole.
- The stroke volume falls and, therefore, the end-diastolic volume rises.
- The lung compliance falls as congestion of the pulmonary capillaries makes the lungs stiffer.
- The decrease in venous return on standing may reduce pulmonary congestion and actually relieve dyspnoea.

2.113   Answer: C

Lack of oxygen will result in anaerobic glycolysis and lactic acid formation.

Heart failure will result in stagnant hypoxia caused by inadequate tissue blood flow.

High altitude will result in respiratory alkalosis.

Hypoxia in *smokers* is the result of the carbon monoxide content of the smoke.

2.114   Answer: D

Pain:

- The blood pressure may fall because of the fall in vascular resistance.
- The heart rate may fall as a result of an increase in cardiac vagal tone.
- Sympathetic cholinergic nerves are motor to the sweat glands.
- The vomiting centre is in the medulla.
- Severe pain will increase cortisol secretion.

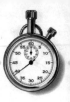

2.115 All are features of haemolytic anaemia except:

☐ A Raised serum bilirubin.

☐ B Increased urinary urobilinogen.

☐ C Increased faecal stercobilinogen.

☐ D Increased serum haptoglobins.

☐ E Reticulocytosis.

2.116 Which statement is false with regard to platelet concentrates?

☐ A Platelet transfusion should be avoided in autoimmune thrombocytopenic purpura.

☐ B Platelets express HLA class 1 antigens but not class 2.

☐ C The platelet count increases by around 10% in pregnancy.

☐ D In massive haemorrhage the platelet count should be kept above 50×10^9.

☐ E Platelet transfusions are contraindicated in heparin-induced thrombocytopenia.

2.117 After a single episode of acute blood loss, which is the most accurate statement?

☐ A The haemoglobin and packed cell volume remain normal for up to 4 h.

☐ B After 4 h, the plasma volume falls.

☐ C The reticulocyte response lasts 24 h.

☐ D There is a fall in neutrophils and platelets initially.

☐ E Clinical assessment is not important until losses are > 750 ml.

2.118 Erythropoietin is raised in which of the following conditions?

☐ A Anaemia.

☐ B Chronic renal failure.

☐ C Cardiac failure.

☐ D High altitude.

☐ E Emphysema.

2.115 Answer: D

Serum haptoglobins are absent because the haptoglobins become saturated with haemoglobin, and the complex is removed by the reticuloendothelial cells.

2.116 Answer: C

Platelet transfusion should be avoided in autoimmune thrombocytopenic purpura, unless there is haemorrhage.

The platelet count typically falls by 10% in pregnancy.

2.117 Answer: A

After a single episode of *blood loss* the haemoglobin and packed cell volume remain normal for up to 4 h because there is initial vasoconstriction with a reduction in blood volume.

After 4 h, however, the plasma volume expands whereas the haemoglobin and packed cell volume fall. There is a rise in neutrophils and platelets.

The reticulocyte response begins on the second or third day and lasts 8–10 days.

The haemoglobin begins to rise by about the seventh day, but if iron stores are depleted this may not rise to normal.

2.118 Answer: B

The stimulus to *erythropoietin* production is low oxygen tension in the tissues of the kidneys.

Erythropoietin levels are low in renal disease and polycythaemia rubra vera.

2.119 One answer is correct. An independence of the P waves and the QRS complexes of the ECG indicate:

    A An early repolarisation of ventricular fibres.

    B A failure of the atrioventricular (AV) node to conduct.

    C A depression of the sinoatrial node.

    D Slowing of conduction at the AV node.

    E A conduction block in the left bundle branch.

2.120 Increased pressure within the carotid sinus causes all of the following except:

    A A decrease in sympathetic tone to arterioles.

    B A decrease in aortic pressure.

    C Reflex bradycardia.

    D Vasodilatation of arterioles.

    E Atrial tachycardia.

2.121 The greatest pressure drop in the circulation occurs across the arterioles because:

    A They have the greatest surface area.

    B They have the greatest cross-sectional area.

    C The velocity of blood flow through them is highest.

    D The velocity of blood flow through them is lowest.

    E They have the greatest resistance.

2.122 Which is false? Carbon dioxide in blood:

    A Is more soluble than oxygen.

    B Is carried in combination with plasma.

    C Is carried mainly as bicarbonate ions.

    D Is hydrated mainly in the red blood cells.

    E Is transported mainly in the red blood cells.

2.119   Answer: B

An independence of the P waves and the QRS complexes of the ECG indicate a failure of the atrioventricular (AV) node to conduct.

2.120   Answer: E

Increased pressure within the carotid sinus does not cause atrial tachycardia.

2.121   Answer: E

The greatest pressure drop in the circulation occurs across the arterioles because they have the greatest resistance.

2.122   Answer: E

Two-thirds of CO_2 is transported in the plasma as bicarbonate ions. As the plasma contains no carbonic anhydrase, the CO_2 is hydrated mainly in the red blood cells. Once formed the bicarbonate diffuses out of the red cells in exchange for chloride ions.

2.123 The urine volume flow rate times the urine concentration of a substance is equal to its rate of:

- [ ] **A** Net tubular secretion.
- [ ] **B** Excretion.
- [ ] **C** Filtration.
- [ ] **D** Net tubular reabsorption.
- [ ] **E** Net active tubular secretion.

2.124 The primary active step for sodium reabsorption in the proximal tubule involves:

- [ ] **A** Na^+/glucose co-transport across the luminal membrane.
- [ ] **B** Na^+/H^+ counter-transport across the luminal membrane.
- [ ] **C** Na^+ transport via the Na^+/K^+ ATPase at the basolateral membrane.
- [ ] **D** Na^+/amino acid co-transport across the luminal membrane.
- [ ] **E** Cl^--coupled Na^+ movement between the cells.

2.125 Pathological features of Crohn's disease include:

- [ ] **A** Not usually affecting the muscularis mucosa.
- [ ] **B** Pseudopolyps.
- [ ] **C** Fistulation.
- [ ] **D** Metaplasia.
- [ ] **E** Shallow ulcers.

2.126 An extraintestinal manifestation of inflammatory bowel disease (IBD) related to disease activity is:

- [ ] **A** Bile duct carcinoma.
- [ ] **B** Cirrhosis.
- [ ] **C** Mouth ulcers.
- [ ] **D** Amyloidosis.
- [ ] **E** Chronic active hepatitis.

2.123 Answer: B

Excretion of a substance always refers to the amount removed from the body.

The amount removed from the body can, in turn, be calculated by multiplying the amount of urine excreted during the time being considered (the volume flow rate) by the concentration per unit volume.

2.124 Answer: C

Sodium transport via the Na^+/K^+ ATPase at the basolateral membrane is the only *transport step for Na^+* in the proximal tubule that involves the direct input of energy to move Na^+ against its electrochemical gradient.

2.125 Answer: C

In *Crohn's* disease the whole thickness of the bowel wall is affected.

Fistulation is common in Crohn's disease, whereas metaplasia and dysplasia can be severe and predispose to carcinoma in ulcerative colitis. Small shallow ulcers are typical in *ulcerative colitis*.

2.126 Answer: C

Other features of IBD related to disease activity include:

- Pyoderma gangrenosum
- Iritis
- Erythema nodosum
- Activity-related arthritis of large joints.

2.127 Which is NOT a feature of Peutz–Jegher polyps?

☐ **A** They are associated with pigmentation around the lips.

☐ **B** They are hamartomas.

☐ **C** They are most common in the small intestine.

☐ **D** Polyps are often present in childhood.

☐ **E** They have a high-grade malignant potential.

2.128 The following statement about CO_2 transport in the blood is true:

☐ **A** High levels of carbonic anhydrase in the plasma allow the plasma to carry more CO_2 than the red blood cell.

☐ **B** Deoxygenated haemoglobin has an increased ability to form carbamino compounds with CO_2.

☐ **C** The high solubility of CO_2 in the plasma allows the plasma to carry more CO_2 than the red blood cells.

☐ **D** The formation of carbamino compounds in the plasma allows the plasma to carry more CO_2 than the red blood cell.

☐ **E** CO_2 is mostly transported in the red blood cells.

2.129 Which is false?

☐ **A** Loop diuretics inhibit the $Na^+/K^+/2Cl^-$ transporter.

☐ **B** Acetazolamide inhibits carbonic anhydrase.

☐ **C** Thiazide diuretics inhibit the Na^+/K^+ co-transporter in the distal tubule.

☐ **D** Mannitol is a freely filtered osmotically active substance that is not reabsorbed and opposes water reabsorption.

☐ **E** Spironolactone is an antagonist of aldosterone.

2.127 Answer: E

Peutz–Jegher polyps have a low-grade malignant potential.

2.128 Answer: B

There is little plasma *carbonic anhydrase*. It is a red cell enzyme.

Similarly, carbamino compounds are formed predominately in the red cells (haemoglobin) and not in the plasma.

Dissolved CO_2 accounts for little of the total CO_2 in the blood. Thus, the correct answer is the *Haldane effect*.

Deoxygenated haemoglobin has an increased ability to bind with CO_2 to form carbamino compounds (ie take up CO_2 in the tissue). When oxygenated in the lung the haemoglobin then gives up CO_2, thus effecting net transport from the tissue to the alveoli. This is the Haldane effect and is physiologically important in gas transport.

2.129 Answer: C

Mannitol is an osmotically active substance that is filtered in the glomerulus and directly opposes water reabsorption from the tubules by the osmotic effect that it exerts there.

Acetazolamide inhibits carbonic anhydrase and so inhibits the reabsorption of bicarbonate. The osmotic effect of the excess bicarbonate in the tubules then opposes water reabsorption.

Loop diuretics inhibit the $Na^+/K^+/2Cl^-$ transporter in the loop of Henle.

Thiazide diuretics inhibit the Na^+/Cl^- co-transporter in the distal tubule.

Aldosterone promotes ENaC transporter channel activity, so *spironolactone*, which is a direct antagonist of aldosterone, has the effect, similar to amiloride, of reducing the activity of the ENaC.

2.130 In a patient with renal failure, which of the following suggests chronic rather than acute renal failure?

- [ ] **A** Microscopic haematuria.
- [ ] **B** Renal bone disease.
- [ ] **C** Normal-sized kidneys on ultrasonography.
- [ ] **D** Pulmonary oedema.
- [ ] **E** Metabolic acidosis.

2.130 Answer: B

The main features that distinguish chronic from acute renal failure are:

- The presence of small kidneys on ultrasonography or other imaging
- The presence of complications of chronic renal failure.

Such complications include:

- Renal bone disease
- A *normochromic/normocytic* anaemia caused by erythropoietin deficiency.

Anaemia can occur in acute renal failure, so it is not diagnostic.

In chronic renal failure, there is:

- a high PTH level
- a high phosphate level
- a low Ca^{2+} level (features of secondary hyperparathyroidism).

Occasionally, tertiary hyperparathyroidism occurs and the high PTH level is able to push the plasma Ca^{2+} level to above normal.

The usual complications of acute renal failure, such as:

- hyperkalaemia
- metabolic acidosis
- pulmonary oedema

can also occur in chronic renal failure.

Haematuria can occur as a result of bleeding within the kidneys, especially intraglomerular bleeding or bleeding from the urinary tract, and does not distinguish between acute and chronic disease.

2.131 **In a patient with anaemia (Hb 8 g/dl) and normal lung function, which statement is true?**

- [ ] **A** Arterial Po_2 is reduced.
- [ ] **B** Arterial–venous O_2 concentration difference is increased.
- [ ] **C** Arterial O_2 saturation is reduced.
- [ ] **D** Po_2 of mixed venous blood is reduced.
- [ ] **E** Cardiac output decreases.

2.132 **In normal renal function which statement is false?**

- [ ] **A** K^+ excretion balances most of the K^+ intake.
- [ ] **B** Along the proximal tubule the K^+ concentration remains nearly equal to that in plasma.
- [ ] **C** Along the descending limb of the loop of Henle, K^+ is reabsorbed via $Na^+/K^+/2Cl^-$ co-transport.
- [ ] **D** Along the distal tubule the net secretion of K^+ is stimulated by aldosterone.
- [ ] **E** Regulation of renal excretion of K^+ in the collecting duct is mostly by changes in the rate of K^+ secretion.

2.131 Answer: D

A patient with *anaemia* and normal lungs typically has a normal arterial Po_2.

If the oxygen consumption and cardiac output are normal, the arterial–venous O_2 concentration difference will also be normal.

Cardiac output can be increased in anaemia and, if this occurs, the arterial–venous O_2 concentration difference will be decreased.

Although, the arterial Po_2 is typically normal, the Po_2 of mixed venous blood must fall. This is because the venous oxygen concentration falls to a very low level as the normal amount of oxygen is extracted, and thus the venous Po_2 is abnormally low.

2.132 Answer: C

Along the *proximal tubule* the K^+ concentration remains almost equal to that in plasma.

As the proximal collecting tubule reabsorbs about two-thirds of the filtrate water, it also reabsorbs about two-thirds (66%) of the filtered K^+.

Along the *descending limb of the loop of Henle*, K^+ is secreted into the tubule lumen from the interstitium.

Along the *thick ascending limb*, K^+ is reabsorbed via $Na^+/K^+/2Cl^-$ co-transport.

In the loop, there is net K^+ reabsorption of 25% of the filtered K^+.

Along the *distal tubule* and *collecting ducts*, there is net secretion of K^+ that is stimulated by aldosterone, and dietary K^+ excess.

Secretion decreases and becomes net reabsorption in K^+ deficiency. Regulation of renal K^+ excretion is in the collecting ducts and is controlled mainly by changes in the rate of K^+ secretion.

2.133 Flow rate through blood vessels:

  A Is directly proportional to the pressure gradient.

  B Is proportional to vascular resistance.

  C Is dependent on the surface area.

  D Is inversely proportional to the pressure gradient.

  E A, B and C above are correct.

2.134 A 23-year-old woman experiences watery diarrhoea, nausea, vomiting, and abdominal cramps 4 hours after eating a chicken sandwich with salad in a restaurant. The most likely organism causing her disease is:

  A *Vibrio vulnificus.*

  B *Listeria monocytogenes.*

  C *Yersinia enterocolitica.*

  D *Clostridium botulinum.*

  E *Staphylococcus aureus.*

2.135 Which one is the most likely biochemical marker of obesity?

  A Mutation of insulin receptor.

  B Decreased serum leptin.

  C Increased blood glucose.

  D Insulin resistance.

  E Increase in C-peptide.

2.136 Erythropoietin is secreted by:

  A Cells in the macula densa.

  B Cells in the proximal tubules.

  C Cells in the distal tubules.

  D Juxtaglomerular cells.

  E Cells in the peritubular capillary bed.

2.133 Answer: A

Flow rate through blood vessels is:

- directly proportional to the pressure gradient
- inversely proportional to vascular resistance.

Flow = Difference in pressure/resistance.

2.134 Answer: E

Staphylococcal food poisoning is manifested 2–6 h after eating food (salad, potato salads) contaminated by a preformed enterotoxin.

Yersinia species is most commonly associated with the ingestion of improperly cooked meat, but symptoms generally begin more than 1 day after ingestion of the contaminated food.

L. monocytogenes symptoms also occur more than 24 h after the ingestion of contaminated foods (milk, ice cream and poultry).

V. vulnificus-associated food poisoning presents usually 24–48 h after the ingestion of contaminated seafood (usually oysters).

2.135 Answer: B

The *leptin* gene is expressed only in adipose tissue and the recessively inherited *ob/ob* obesity in mice. Both copies of the gene are defective because of the presence of a stop cordon that truncates the protein at amino acid 105. Treatment of obese mice with leptin reduces food intake and body fat.

2.136 Answer: E

Erythropoietin is secreted by cells in the paritubular capillary bed.

2.137 Most absorption of short chain fatty acids produced by bacteria occurs in:

- [ ] **A** The jejunum.
- [ ] **B** The colon.
- [ ] **C** The ileum.
- [ ] **D** The stomach.
- [ ] **E** The caecum.

2.138 When the radius of the resistance vessels is increased, which of the following is also increased?

- [ ] **A** Systolic blood pressure.
- [ ] **B** Viscosity of the blood.
- [ ] **C** Haematocrit.
- [ ] **D** Capillary blood flow.
- [ ] **E** Blood pH.

2.139 The symptoms of the dumping syndrome are caused in part by:

- [ ] **A** Increased blood pressure.
- [ ] **B** Reduced blood pressure.
- [ ] **C** Increased CCK secretion.
- [ ] **D** Iron deficiency anaemia.
- [ ] **E** Rapid entry of food or liquid into the small intestine.

2.140 Which is false with regard to brown fat?

- [ ] **A** It is more abundant in children than in adults.
- [ ] **B** It is richer in mitochondria than normal fat.
- [ ] **C** It is more vascular than normal fat.
- [ ] **D** It can generate more heat when parasympathetic nerves are stimulated.
- [ ] **E** It is more important in infants than shivering.

2.137   Answer: B

Most absorption of short chain fatty acids produced by bacteria occurs in the colon.

2.138   Answer: D

When the radius of the resistance vessels is increased, capillary blood flow is also increased.

2.139   Answer: E

The principal cause of this syndrome is the rapid entry of hypertonic meals into the intestine, resulting in large volumes of water entering into the gut and, hence, hypovolaemia.

The rapid absorption of glucose from the intestine and the resultant hyperglycaemia cause the abrupt rise in insulin secretion.

Therefore, patients who have had *gastric surgery* (either post-gastrectomy or after surgery where part of the stomach has been removed or anastomosed to the jejunum) may develop hypoglycaemic symptoms after meals.

2.140   Answer: D

Metabolic activity in *brown fat* is stimulated by sympathetic activity.

It is richer in mitochondria, has a higher metabolic rate and is, therefore, more vascular than normal fat. Infants do not shiver well.

3. PATHOLOGY

Multiple true/false questions

3.1   **Meckel's diverticulum:**

☐ **A** Is a remnant of the vitello-intestinal duct.

☐ **B** Occurs in 0.2% of patients.

☐ **C** Is found on the anti-mesenteric border of the terminal ileum.

☐ **D** May contain ectopic colonic mucosa.

☐ **E** May present with intussusception.

3.2   **Intussusception:**

☐ **A** Is most common in boys aged from 1 to 6 months.

☐ **B** Is associated with pyloric stenosis.

☐ **C** Rarely presents with vomiting.

☐ **D** Demonstrates the classic 'doughnut' sign on ultrasonography.

☐ **E** May be palpable on abdominal examination.

3.3   **A keratoacanthoma:**

☐ **A** Is usually a self-healing lesion.

☐ **B** Histologically resembles squamous cell carcinoma cells.

☐ **C** Histologically resembles basal cell carcinoma cells.

☐ **D** Is malignant.

☐ **E** Contains eosinophilic inclusion bodies.

3.4   **Seborrhoeic keratoses:**

☐ **A** Are benign.

☐ **B** Are deeply pigmented.

☐ **C** Are more likely to occur on the trunk.

☐ **D** Are usually associated with infection.

☐ **E** Are caused by a proliferation of epidermal cells.

3.1 Answer: A, E

Occurs in 2% of patients, is 2 cm long and located 2 feet (0.6 m) from the ileocaecal junction. Usually an incidental finding at laparotomy but may result in rectal bleeding (caused by ectopic gastric mucosa), umbilical discharge, small bowel volvulus or intussusception.

3.2 Answer: D, E

Intussusception results when a segment of bowel invaginates into an adjacent segment. It is most common in boys aged 3 months to 2 years. A seasonal incidence has been described, with peaks in the spring, summer and middle of winter. Red-currant jelly stool is a typical finding, and there may well be a palpable mass on abdominal or per rectum examination. Ultrasonography demonstrates the classic 'doughnut' sign or 'target' sign, with hypoechoic, oedematous surrounding bowel representing the intussuscepiens, and the central more echogenic, invaginated bowel representing the intussusceptum.

3.3 Answer: A, B

This is a round, firm, usually flesh-coloured nodule with sharply sloping borders and a characteristic central crater containing keratinous material.

Onset is rapid – usually within 1 or 2 months the lesion reaches its full size. Common sites are sun-exposed areas, the face, the forearm and the dorsum of the hand. Spontaneous involution usually starts within a few months. This lesion is sometimes difficult to differentiate clinically and histologically from squamous cell carcinoma. If the diagnosis is uncertain, a lengthwise through-and-through midline or total excisional biopsy should be done. Eosinophilic inclusion bodies are found in molluscum contagiosum.

3.4 Answer: A, B, C, E

These are benign lesions also known as basal cell papillomas. They usually occur on the trunk and their incidence increases from age 40 onwards. They are not associated with infection.

3.5   **With regard to diathermy:**

☐ **A**   The electrical frequency produced is in the range 50–250 kHz.

☐ **B**   The current passes through the patient when using bipolar diathermy.

☐ **C**   Cutting is produced by a continuous current.

☐ **D**   Coagulation uses a square waveform.

☐ **E**   Spirit-based skin preparations should be avoided.

3.6   **In gas gangrene:**

☐ **A**   The patient's gut flora may be the source of infection.

☐ **B**   *Clostridium septicum* may be responsible.

☐ **C**   Prophylaxis with benzylpenicillin may be used in high-risk groups.

☐ **D**   Pain is often out of proportion to clinical findings.

☐ **E**   Definitive treatment is with antibiotics.

3.7   **Risk factors for MRSA (methicillin-resistant *Staphylococcus aureus*) colonisation include:**

☐ **A**   An ITU (intensive therapy unit) stay.

☐ **B**   Female gender.

☐ **C**   The presence of an indwelling device.

☐ **D**   Chronic medical illness.

☐ **E**   Prolonged hospitalisation.

3.8   **In sickle cell anaemia:**

☐ **A**   HbS is less soluble than HbA.

☐ **B**   Inheritance is autosomal recessive.

☐ **C**   Preoperative exchange transfusion is usually required.

☐ **D**   Opiates should be avoided.

☐ **E**   Patients have chronic haemolytic anaemia with high reticulocyte counts.

3.5   Answer: C, D, E

The electrical frequency produced is between 300 kHz and 3 MHz. The current passes through the patient in monopolar diathermy only. Coagulation is produced by interrupted pulses of current and a square waveform. Cutting is produced by a continuous sine wave current.

3.6   Answer: A, B, C, D

The organisms responsible are *Clostridium* species (*C. septicum*, *C. oedmatiens* and *C. perfringens*). Contamination may occur from the patient's faecal flora.

Definitive treatment is surgical debridement.

3.7   Answer: A, C, D, E

Males are more at risk.

3.8   Answer: A, B, E

Normal haemoglobin has two α and two β chains. In sickle cell disease single amino acid substitution occurs on the β chain whereby valine is substituted for glutamic acid at position 6. The resulting HbS is less soluble than HbA. The sickle haemoglobin gene is inherited as autosomal recessive. It is commonly seen in patients of African–Caribbean descent. When deoxygenated haemoglobin undergoes polymerisation and forms characteristic sickle cells, blockage of small vessels results in vaso-occlusive events. Sickling may be precipitated by infection, fever, dehydration, cold or hypoxia. Patients with complications should be treated with oxygen, intravenous fluids and analgesia (often opiates). Exchange transfusions are rarely required preoperatively.

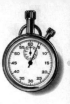

3.9 **A tourniquet:**

☐ **A** Should not be inflated to more than 100 mmHg above diastolic blood pressure.

☐ **B** Should not be used continuously for more than 90 min.

☐ **C** May result in myoglobinuria.

☐ **D** May result in neuropraxia.

☐ **E** May result in decreased blood viscosity.

3.10 **With regard to surgical wounds:**

☐ **A** An elective hemicolectomy wound is regarded as contaminated.

☐ **B** A hernia repair wound is regarded as clean.

☐ **C** An intraperitoneal abscess produces a clean-contaminated wound.

☐ **D** The infection rate for a clean wound is 1–2%.

☐ **E** The infection rate for a dirty wound is 20–25%.

3.11 **When sterilising equipment:**

☐ **A** Ethylene oxide is used for heat-sensitive items.

☐ **B** Autoclaving relies on the presence of steam.

☐ **C** Alcohols are highly effective against viruses.

☐ **D** Glutaraldehyde will not kill spores.

☐ **E** Gamma irradiation is used in industry.

3.12 **With regard to hepatitis B:**

☐ **A** It is a double-stranded DNA virus.

☐ **B** HBs antigen is the first indicator of infection.

☐ **C** HBe antigen is a marker of infectivity.

☐ **D** Liver cirrhosis is a risk of chronic infection.

☐ **E** Immunisation confers protection for 10 years.

3.9   Answer: B, C, D

Tourniquets should not be inflated to more than 100 mmHg above systolic blood pressure.

Their use may result in increased blood viscosity.

3.10   Answer: B, D

Hernia repair (no viscus opened): clean wound with an infection rate of 1–2%.

An intraperitoneal abscess: dirty wound with an infection rate of 40%.

An elective right hemicolectomy wound is regarded as clean contaminated with an infection rate of 5–10%.

A clean contaminated wound has an infection rate of < 10%.

3.11   Answer: A, B, E

Alcohols and other chemical disinfectants are not equally active against all micro-organisms. Mycobacteria and slow viruses are resistant whereas Gram-positive bacteria are very sensitive.

Glutaraldehyde is a widely used sporicide.

3.12   Answer: B, C, D

Hepatitis B is a single-stranded DNA virus and is transmitted by inoculation, sexual contact or vertical transmission. All medical staff should be immunised and protection is conferred for up to 5 years.

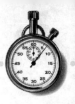

3.13   Which of the following are clinical signs that indicate the development of malignant melanoma from a benign naevus?

☐ **A**   Change in shape.

☐ **B**   Change in size.

☐ **C**   Bleeding.

☐ **D**   Sensory changes.

☐ **E**   Diameter > 7 mm.

3.14   Bladder cancer:

☐ **A**   Mostly presents with painful haematuria.

☐ **B**   In the UK is usually an adenocarcinoma.

☐ **C**   Is associated with schistosomiasis infection.

☐ **D**   Is associated with exposure to aniline dyes.

☐ **E**   Spreads preferentially to the iliac and para-aortic lymph nodes.

3.15   With regard to rapid sequence induction:

☐ **A**   It may be used in emergency trauma situation.

☐ **B**   Pressure over the cricoid cartilage may reduce aspiration.

☐ **C**   Induction agents need to be highly water soluble.

☐ **D**   Thiopentone may cause myocardial depression.

☐ **E**   Propofol may cause hypotension.

3.16   Perioperatively:

☐ **A**   Ulnar nerve lesions may be caused by placing the arms in supination.

☐ **B**   Excessive external rotation may cause a brachial plexus injury.

☐ **C**   The lithotomy position may cause tibial nerve injury.

☐ **D**   Radial nerve injury may be caused by a tourniquet.

☐ **E**   Neuropraxias spontaneously recover in 90% of cases.

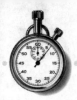

3.13 Answer: all true

Major signs include change in colour, size or shape, or a diameter > 7 mm. Minor signs include bleeding, sensory changes or inflammation.

3.14 Answer: C, D, E

Of cases of bladder cancer, 80% present with painless haematuria. In the UK transitional cell carcinoma is the most common but, worldwide, schistosomiasis infection is implicated in squamous cell carcinoma. Chlorinate hydrocarbons, aniline dyes and smoking are risk factors.

3.15 Answer: A, B, D, E

Induction agents need to be highly lipid soluble to cross the blood–brain barrier rapidly.

3.16 Answer: B, D, E

Ulnar nerve lesions are prevented by placing the patient's arms in supination. The lithotomy position may cause fibular/peroneal nerve injury and may be prevented by adequately padding the lithotomy poles.

3.17 **Tetanus:**

☐ **A** Is a Gram-negative rod.

☐ **B** Exerts its effects via an endotoxin.

☐ **C** Acts postsynaptically.

☐ **D** Is destroyed by autoclaving.

☐ **E** Can be treated definitively with benzylpenicillin.

3.18 **Which of the following may cause toxic megacolon?**

☐ **A** Ulcerative colitis.

☐ **B** Crohn's disease.

☐ **C** *Yersinia* spp.

☐ **D** Radiation colitis.

☐ **E** Pseudomembranous colitis.

3.19 **In pseudomembranous colitis:**

☐ **A** The causative organism is a Gram-positive anaerobe.

☐ **B** Broad-spectrum antibiotics are implicated.

☐ **C** Asymptomatic carriers should be treated.

☐ **D** Vancomycin is a second-line therapy.

☐ **E** Epithelial necrosis may occur.

3.20 **Which of the following are true?**

☐ **A** Atrophy results from a reduction in cell numbers.

☐ **B** Dysplasia is often premalignant.

☐ **C** Barrett's oesophagus is an example of hypertrophy.

☐ **D** Hyperplasia is an increase in cell size.

☐ **E** Cervical cancer is preceded by dysplasia.

3.21 **With regard to radiotherapy:**

☐ **A** The response of tissues depends on the degree of differentiation.

☐ **B** Cells in the resting phase are most vulnerable.

☐ **C** It may be used alone as a curative treatment for some cancers.

☐ **D** It may cause mucositis.

☐ **E** Acute toxicity is seen within minutes.

3.17 Answer: all false

Tetanus is caused by the Gram-positive, spore-forming rod, *Clostridium tetani*. Its exotoxin acts at the presynaptic terminals of inhibitory nerves. The extotoxin is relatively resistant to autoclaving.

Management involves the use of IV benzylpenicillin, wound debridement and ITU support, but mortality is about 50% in spite of this.

3.18 Answer: all true

Toxic megacolon is a potentially lethal condition. It is defined as a colonic dilatation > 6 cm accompanied by signs of systemic toxicity.

3.19 Answer: A, B, D, E

In severe infection epithelial necrosis may occur forming a pseudomembrane.

Asymptomatic carriers do not require treatment.

3.20 Answer: A, B, E

Atrophy is a reduction in cell size or number. Barrett's oesophagus is an example of metaplasia, where squamous epithelium is replaced by columnar epithelium. Hyperplasia describes cell proliferation.

3.21 Answer: A, C, D

Radiotherapy is most effective against cells that are poorly differentiated and/or rapidly dividing cells. It may be used as a curative treatment, e.g. in squamous cell carcinoma of the skin, as well as for palliative or adjuvant therapy. Acute toxicity occurs within days and may include mucositis.

3.22 Which of the following tumours and tumour markers are correctly paired?

☐ **A** CEA and colon cancer.

☐ **B** β-hCG (β-human chorionic gonadotrophin) and choriocarcinoma.

☐ **C** *BRCA*-1 and breast cancer.

☐ **D** CA-19.9 and ovarian cancer.

☐ **E** α-Fetoprotein (AFP) and hepatoma.

3.23 The following may be seen in acute renal failure:

☐ **A** Hyponatraemia.

☐ **B** Hypokalaemia.

☐ **C** Urinary sodium < 20 mmol/l.

☐ **D** Hypercalcaemia.

☐ **E** Metabolic acidosis.

3.24 The following are diagnostic features of the systemic inflammatory response (SIRS):

☐ **A** Temperature < 36°C.

☐ **B** Heart rate < 60 beats/min (bpm).

☐ **C** Respiratory rate > 15 bpm.

☐ **D** White cell count (WCC) < 4000/mm^3.

☐ **E** Pao_2 < 8 Pa.

3.25 In HIV infection:

☐ **A** The first symptoms usually occur within 3 months of infection.

☐ **B** Generalised persistent lymphadenopathy may follow seroconversion.

☐ **C** CD8 lymphocyte counts are used as a marker of disease activity.

☐ **D** Invasive cervical carcinoma is an indicator disease for AIDS.

☐ **E** Treatment involves peroxidase inhibitors.

3.22 Answer: A, B, E

BRCA-1 is a tumour-suppressor gene involved in breast cancer. CA-19.9 is associated with pancreatic cancer. CEA (carcinoembryonic antigen) is associated with pancreatic, colon and stomach cancer.

3.23 Answer: A, C, E

Prerenal failure will cause a urinary sodium < 20 mmol/l. Other abnormalities include hyponatraemia, hyperkalaemia, hypocalcaemia and a metabolic acidosis.

3.24 Answer: A, D

SIRS requires at least two of the following:

- Temperature > 38°C or < 36°C
- Heart rate > 90 bpm
- Respiratory rate > 20 bpm or $Paco_2$ > 4.3 kPa
- WCC > 12 000 or < 4000/mm^3.

3.25 Answer: B, D

The first 3 months after HIV (human immunodeficiency virus) infection are typically free of symptoms. Acute seroconversion illness may accompany seroconversion and generalised persistent lymphadenopathy may follow.

CD4 counts are used in disease monitoring. There are a large number of indicator diseases for acquired immune deficiency syndrome (AIDS) including invasive cervical cancer.

Treatment involves reverse transcriptase and protease inhibitors.

3.26 **With regard to pneumonia:**

- A Lobar pneumonia is usually caused by *Haemophilus influenzae*.
- B Lobar pneumonia usually occurs in otherwise healthy individuals.
- C Untreated bronchopneumonia may result in lung fibrosis.
- D Lobar pneumonia may affect several lobes at a time.
- E Pneumococci spread via the pores of Kohn.

3.27 **Side effects of steroids include:**

- A Pancreatitis.
- B Avascular necrosis.
- C Bone marrow suppression.
- D Hyperkalaemia.
- E Osteoporosis.

3.28 **Thrombocytopenia may be seen in:**

- A Massive blood transfusions.
- B Aplastic anaemia.
- C Carcinomatosis.
- D Disseminated intravascular coagulation.
- E After splenectomy.

3.29 **Wilms' tumours:**

- A Are tumours of primitive nephroblastic tissues.
- B Are the most common genitourinary malignancy in children.
- C Usually present with haematuria.
- D Unilaterally have a cure rate of 90%.
- E Rarely invade locally.

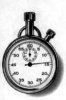

3.26 Answer: B, C, D, E

Lobar pneumonia usually occurs in otherwise healthy young adults and is caused by *Streptococcus pneumoniae* in the vast majority of cases. Bronchopneumonia occurs where immunity has been reduced such as in elderly or immunocompromised individuals. It is more likely to heal with fibrosis unlike lobar pneumonia, which may heal spontaneously without antibiotics. Pneumococci are thought to spread between the alveoli through the pores of Kohn.

3.27 Answer: A, B, E

Steroids side effects include osteoporosis, avascular necrosis of bone, hypertension, hypernatraemia, hypokalaemia, water retention, diabetes, Cushing's syndrome and obesity. Bone marrow suppression may be seen with azathioprine.

3.28 Answer: A, B, C, D

Thrombocytopenia most commonly arises from the destruction of platelets in the periphery. It may also be seen after heparin therapy and in immune thrombocytopenia as well as after chemotherapy.

Thrombocytosis is commonly seen after splenectomy.

3.29 Answer: A, B, D, E

Wilms' tumours usually show differentiation towards the embryonal kidney, and 50% occur before the age of 3 years. They usually present with a mass; haematuria, loin pain and hypertension are uncommon.

There is an 80–90% cure rate with surgery and chemotherapy. They invade locally and may spread to the adrenals, liver and paraspinal region.

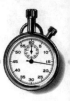

3.30 **Transitional cell carcinoma of the bladder:**

- A Accounts for 80% of lower urinary tract tumours.
- B Is a superficial/low-grade papillary tumour in 80% of cases.
- C Is common where schistosomiasis is endemic.
- D Has a tumour grade that is the single most important prognostic factor.
- E Has grade 3 tumours that display marked cellular atypia.

3.31 **Bone and soft tissue tumours:**

- A There is a bimodal age-specific incidence rate of bone sarcomas.
- B Ionising radiation is a recognised cause of sarcomas.
- C Liposarcomas affect the elderly population.
- D Ewing's sarcoma typically occurs at the epiphysis.
- E Osteosarcoma typically occurs at the metaphysis.

3.32 **Predisposing factors for renal cell carcinoma include:**

- A Osler–Weber–Rendu syndrome.
- B Von Hippel–Lindau disease.
- C Smoking.
- D Chronic haemodialysis.
- E Cadmium exposure.

3.33 **Squamous cell carcinoma of the oesophagus:**

- A Is the most prevalent form of oesophageal cancer in developing countries.
- B In western countries is predominantly an adenocarcinoma.
- C Strongly implicates alcohol and tobacco.
- D Has been associated with the human papillomavirus.
- E Has an aetiology involving Epstein–Barr virus (EBV).

3.30 Answer: A, B, E

Schistosomiasis causes squamous cell carcinoma of the bladder. It is the depth of invasion that is the single most important prognostic factor.

3.31 Answer: A, B, C, E

Ewing's sarcoma occurs more commonly at the diaphyses.

3.32 Answer: B, C, D, E

Risk factors for renal cell carcinoma include increased age, male sex, smoking, obesity, long-term dialysis and several genetic syndromes, including familial clear cell carcinoma, von Hippel–Lindau syndrome and tuberous sclerosis. Exposure to asbestos, petroleum products and dry cleaning agents appears to increase the risk. Cadmium and organic solvents are also implicated.

3.33 Answer: A, B, C, D

Squamous cell carcinoma of the oesophagus is more strongly associated with smoking and increased alcohol intake than oesophageal adenocarcinomas or gastric cancer. Reflux is also a risk factor for the development of adenocarcinoma via Barrett's metaplasia. There is no evidence to date that the EBV is implicated.

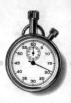

3.34   In lasers:

- [ ] **A** Class 1 lasers are safe to stare into for unlimited periods.
- [ ] **B** Class 4 lasers include all medical lasers.
- [ ] **C** Class 3 lasers are safe within the time of the blink reflex.
- [ ] **D** Class 3 lasers cause blindness after shorter exposure or exposure from mirrored surfaces.
- [ ] **E** Pulsed lasers require lower intensity goggles than continuous wave lasers.

3.35   A high PSA may be found in:

- [ ] **A** Prostatic cancer.
- [ ] **B** Benign prostatic hyperplasia.
- [ ] **C** Recent ejaculation.
- [ ] **D** Prostatic infection.
- [ ] **E** Advancing age.

3.36   In acute retention:

- [ ] **A** Digital rectal examination (DRE) is essential.
- [ ] **B** Stress is a common precipitating cause.
- [ ] **C** It usually supervenes in patients with prostatic obstruction.
- [ ] **D** Routine investigation of the upper tracts is advisable.
- [ ] **E** Failure to void after catheter removal is an indication for further investigation.

3.37   In osteomalacia:

- [ ] **A** There may be a low serum calcium.
- [ ] **B** Patients commonly display symptoms of hypocalcaemia.
- [ ] **C** The pathognomonic feature is Looser's zone.
- [ ] **D** Alkaline phosphatase (ALP) may be raised.
- [ ] **E** Sarcomatous change is common.

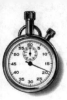

3.34   Answer: A, B, D

Pulsed lasers require more protective goggles than continuous wave lasers.

It is class 2 lasers that are safe within the blink reflex.

3.35   Answer: all true

Prostate-specific antigen (PSA) is also raised after urinary tract instrumentation such as catheterisation. Per rectum examination does not usually cause a significant rise.

3.36   Answer: A, B, C, E

Routine investigation of the upper tracts is not required unless clinical features such as infection/inflammation are present.

3.37   Answer: A, C, D

Sarcomatous change is associated with Paget's disease. Symptoms of hypocalcaemia in osteomalacia are rare.

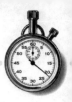

3.38 **Developmental dysplasia of the hip:**

- [ ] **A** Resulting in irreducible dislocation of a neonatal hip is common.
- [ ] **B** Can be diagnosed with Ortolani's test.
- [ ] **C** Can be visualised early by ultrasonography.
- [ ] **D** Will stabilise without treatment in the first 2 weeks of life in many cases.
- [ ] **E** Is more common in the firstborn.

3.39 **Osteoporosis:**

- [ ] **A** Is an inevitable consequence of ageing.
- [ ] **B** Is associated with prolonged immobilisation.
- [ ] **C** Is often associated with a low calcium.
- [ ] **D** Is often associated with a reduced ALP.
- [ ] **E** Is defined by a bone mineral density > 2.5 SD (standard deviation) below the young adult mean.

3.40 **Extradural haemorrhage:**

- [ ] **A** Is almost always caused by trauma.
- [ ] **B** If enlarging typically results in a biconvex mass.
- [ ] **C** Results in accumulation of blood between the skull and dura mater.
- [ ] **D** May result from a torn sagittal sinus.
- [ ] **E** Occurs between the dura and arachnoid mater.

3.41 **Direct spinal cord compression above the conus results in:**

- [ ] **A** Hypotonia.
- [ ] **B** Spastic paraparesis.
- [ ] **C** Extensor plantar response.
- [ ] **D** Clonus.
- [ ] **E** Fasciculations.

3.38 Answer: B, C, D, E

Congenital dysplasia is usually dislocated but reducible.

3.39 Answer: A, B, E

Alkaline phosphatase is usually normal or raised after a fracture.

3.40 Answer: A, B, C, D

Extradural haemorrhage may result from a laceration of the middle meningeal vessels (typically), as well as other meningeal vessels, oozing from the diploë, bone and stripped dura on each side of an associated fracture. The resulting haematoma collects in the space between the skull and the dura mater, raising the intracranial pressure. Factors that affect the evolution of a haematoma include: the volume of cerebrospinal fluid (CSF) that needs to be pushed out before coning begins, the rate of haemorrhage and the age of the victim. The younger the victim, the better the prognosis.

3.41 Answer: B, C, D

Hypertonia is typical. Fasciculations, flaccidity, muscle wasting and absent reflexes are true of lower motor lesions. The conus is at T12–L1. Direct compression above this would result in upper motor signs. Below the conus, only the exiting nerve roots – cauda equina – are affected.

3.42 **Compression of the cauda equina may present as:**

☐ **A** A palpable bladder.

☐ **B** Altered perineal sensation.

☐ **C** Increased anal tone.

☐ **D** Absent ankle jerks.

☐ **E** Bilateral buttock pain.

3.43 **Core biopsy:**

☐ **A** Is more painful than fine-needle aspiration (FNA).

☐ **B** Enables the use of immunohistochemistry and special stains.

☐ **C** Does not usually allow differentiation between ductal carcinoma *in situ* and invasive carcinoma.

☐ **D** Requires local anaesthetic.

☐ **E** Does not result in preservation of tissue architecture.

3.44 **Fine-needle aspiration:**

☐ **A** Requires local anaesthetic.

☐ **B** Can be used on any solid lesion.

☐ **C** Can be useful in the diagnosis of metastases.

☐ **D** Allows differentiation between follicular adenoma and follicular carcinoma.

☐ **E** Does not usually allow determination of tissue architecture.

3.42 Answer: A, B, D, E

The adult spinal cord terminates at the level of vertebrae L1–L2, with the terminal bundle of lumbar and sacral nerve roots within the spinal canal forming the cauda equina below; the nerve roots then separate and exit at their specific foramina. Compression of the cauda equina is most commonly caused by herniation of a disc, often in association with degenerative or congenital spinal stenosis, and can result in cauda equina syndrome (CES). Signs of CES include severe bilateral sciatica, bilateral foot weakness and saddle-type hypaesthesia or anaesthesia in the areas innervated by nerve roots S2–S5, and retention or incontinence of urine, stool or both.

3.43 Answer: A, B, D

Core biopsy allows a formal histological assessment and invasive carcinoma can be differentiated from ductal carcinoma.

3.44 Answer: all true

FNA specimens are usually acquired using 20- to 25-gauge needles and generally provide a sample for cytological examination, whereas needle-core biopsy specimens are obtained using larger 14- to 18-gauge needles and primarily provide a tissue core for histological assessment. Although both techniques are very safe, FNA is often preferred in sampling deeply placed lesions or sites adjacent to major vessels, or in situations in which needles have to be passed through the bowel wall. Cytological samples can be rapidly stained and examined, thereby providing immediate assessment of adequacy, and in many cases a provisional diagnosis can be made while the patient remains in the radiology department. However, FNA is a cytological method that provides no information on tissue structure.

With needle-core biopsy, there is preservation of tissue architecture, which may be important in the assessment and subtyping of some tumours. It is also easier to apply histochemical and immunohistochemical techniques to paraffin wax-embedded biopsy material.

Core biopsy allows a formal histological assessment and invasive carcinoma can be differentiated from ductal carcinoma.

3.45 **Of suture materials:**

　A Polypropylene is often used in abdominal aortic aneurysm repair.

　B Nylon is an appropriate suture material for skin closure.

　C Braided suture materials are ideal in patients with diabetes.

　D Absorbable sutures are best used in the biliary tree.

　E PDS is completely degraded within 30 days.

3.46 **In suture materials:**

　A They are always weakened at the point of a knot.

　B Tensile strength is expressed as the force required to break a suture when the two ends are pulled apart.

　C Catgut is degraded via hydrolysis.

　D Silk is less likely to cause a stitch abscess than Vicryl.

　E Polyglactin (Vicryl) is an absorbable suture.

3.47 **The cellular response to wound healing:**

　A Involves migration of neutrophils, macrophages and lymphocytes.

　B Involves the extracellular matrix containing fibronectin and glycosaminoglycans.

　C Involves maximum collagen production at 2 days.

　D Involves contact inhibition which prevents further epithelial growth.

　E Involves contraction that can account for up to 80% reduction in wound size.

3.48 **For the 'average' 70-kg man:**

　A Total body water is 42 l (about 60% of body weight).

　B There is 14 l in the extracellular compartments.

　C The plasma volume is 3 l.

　D Total body Na^+ is 4200 mmol (50% in extracellular fluid [ECF]).

　E Normal osmolality of ECF is 280–295 mosmol/kg.

3.45 Answer: A, B, D

Nylon (e.g. Ethilon™) is a synthetic monofilament material widely used for skin suture. Braided suture materials have interstices for bacteria to lodge in and are not a first choice in diabetic patients. The biliary tree and urothelium may react to permanent suture material and this may result in stone formation. Polydioxanone (PDS) is a monofilament. It absorbs slowly and there is minimal absorption until about 90 days.

3.46 Answer: A, B, E

Absorbable suture are broken down by either proteolysis (such as catgut) or hydrolysis (e.g. Vicryl, Dexon). Silk is strong and handles well but induces strong tissue reaction. Its capillarity encourages infection, causing suture sinuses and abscesses.

Synthetic suture materials are:

- *Absorbable*:
    - polyglycolic acid (Dexon)
    - polyglactin (Vicryl)
    - PDS
    - polyglyconate (Maxon).
- *Non-absorbable*:
    - polyamide (nylon)
    - polyester (Dacron)
    - polypropylene (Prolene).

3.47 Answer: A, B, D, E

Maximum collagen production occurs at 20–25 days and maximum wound strength at 3–6 months.

3.48 Answer: all true

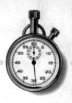

3.49 *Staphylococcus aureus:*

- ☐ **A** Does not produce coagulase.
- ☐ **B** Is the most common agent of osteomyelitis.
- ☐ **C** Is carried asymptomatically in up to 40% of normal people.
- ☐ **D** May cause diarrhoea.
- ☐ **E** May cause toxic shock syndrome.

3.50 *Clostridium* **spp. can produce:**

- ☐ **A** Gas gangrene.
- ☐ **B** Food poisoning.
- ☐ **C** Tetanus.
- ☐ **D** Diarrhoea.
- ☐ **E** Respiratory failure.

3.51 **Anaerobic sepsis:**

- ☐ **A** May result from a gangrenous hernia.
- ☐ **B** Is usually caused by *Bacteroides fragilis* in abdominal surgery.
- ☐ **C** Can be effectively treated with metronidazole.
- ☐ **D** May follow spontaneous bowel perforation.
- ☐ **E** Is susceptible to aminoglycosides.

3.52 **Gout:**

- ☐ **A** Predominantly affects middle-aged men.
- ☐ **B** Is effectively treated with aspirin.
- ☐ **C** May be treated acutely with xanthine oxidase inhibitors.
- ☐ **D** May be caused by low levels of hypoxanthine–guanine–phosphoribosyltransferase (HPGRT).
- ☐ **E** Has clinical features that include kidney stones and tophi.

3.49 Answer: B, C, D, E

This organism produces coagulase that catalyses the production of fibrin from fibrinogen. It spreads by airborne transmission and via the hands of healthcare workers. Coagulase-negative staphylococci are differentiated from *S. aureus* by their inability to produce free plasma coagulase and are often are found among the normal flora of human skin and mucous membranes. Coagulase-negative staphylococci become potentially pathogenic as soon as the natural balance between micro-organisms and the immune system is disturbed: immunocompromised patients are particularly susceptible to intravascular catheter-related infection.

3.50 Answer: all true

Members of the species include:

- *C. difficile*
- *C. perfringens*
- *C. botulinum*
- *C. tetani*.

3.51 Answer: A, B, C, D

Infection with non-sporing anaerobes is endogenous. It usually follows spontaneous bowel perforation or elective surgery and is also commonly seen in sepsis of the female genital tract, often secondary to, septic abortion and complicated caesarean sections. Effective management involves surgery and antibiotics. Almost all anaerobes are susceptible to metronidazole.

3.52 Answer: A, D, E

Xanthine oxidase inhibitors are used for long-term prophylaxis (e.g. allopurinol).

Aspirin causes decreased excretion of uric acid.

3.53 **With regard to the thyroid gland:**

- [ ] **A** Iodine deficiency is rare because of the fortification of table salt.
- [ ] **B** The Guthrie test is useful only in babies born to hypothyroid mothers.
- [ ] **C** Both T_3 (triiodothyronine) and T_4 (thyroxine) have a negative feedback on the hypothalamus and anterior pituitary.
- [ ] **D** The anterior pituitary produces thyroid-releasing hormone (TRH).
- [ ] **E** Thyroid hyperplasia may be a result of high TSH (thyroid-stimulating hormone) levels.

3.54 **Vitamin K:**

- [ ] **A** Is antagonised by warfarin.
- [ ] **B** Needs to be taken in the diet regularly to avoid deficiency.
- [ ] **C** Is a coenzyme for factors III, V, IX and X.
- [ ] **D** Is given to children to treat intracranial haemorrhage.
- [ ] **E** Deficiency may result from long-term antibiotic therapy.

3.55 **In ultrasonography of the biliary tract:**

- [ ] **A** The diameter of the non-obstructed common hepatic duct increases after a cholecystectomy.
- [ ] **B** Gallstones as small as 2 mm in diameter may be detected with an accuracy of 90%.
- [ ] **C** A non-dilated biliary tract excludes the possibility of obstruction.
- [ ] **D** Biliary tract dilatation may precede the onset of clinically detectable jaundice.
- [ ] **E** Ultrasonography is better at assessing stones in the distal portion of the common duct than stones in the proximal portion.

3.56 **Hypocalcaemia results in:**

- [ ] **A** Arrhythmias.
- [ ] **B** Heart failure.
- [ ] **C** Renal stones.
- [ ] **D** Diarrhoea.
- [ ] **E** Muscle weakness.

3.53   Answer: A, C, D, E

The Guthrie test is a neonatal screening test used on all newborn babies looking for raised TSH levels.

3.54   Answer: A, C, E

Vitamin K deficiency is rare because most is synthesised by gut bacteria.

Newborn babies have sterile guts and cannot initially make vitamin K.

Every neonate is given vitamin K to prevent haemorrhagic disease of the newborn, which may result in intracranial haemorrhage.

3.55   Answer: A, B, D

The diameter of the non-obstructed duct increases after cholecystectomy or previous obstruction. Clear bile transmits sound without attenuation, unlike blood, which attenuates the ultrasonic beam.

Dilatation of the biliary tract does not always occur and is less likely if the obstruction is the result of the common duct being encased by tumour, or if the obstruction is recent. Biliary tract dilatation may precede the onset of clinically detectable jaundice and this may occur when only some segments of the intrahepatic biliary tree are affected by tumour or in complete obstruction such as carcinoma of the head of the pancreas.

3.56   Answer: A, B, C, E

Causes of hypocalcaemia include heart failure, arrhythmias, calcification of arteries and renal stones via metastatic calcification. Tiredness, weakness and a sluggish nervous response may also be seen. Constipation rather than diarrhoea is seen.

3.57 **Total parenteral nutrition (TPN):**

- [ ] **A** Is used in preference to enteral nutrition.
- [ ] **B** Is indicated when a patient is eating less than 70% of his or her recommended daily intake.
- [ ] **C** Can be complicated by hyperglycaemia.
- [ ] **D** Can be complicated by infection.
- [ ] **E** Is most commonly administered via a central venous catheter.

3.58 **Wernicke–Korsakoff syndrome:**

- [ ] **A** Causes ataxia.
- [ ] **B** Can lead to short-term memory loss.
- [ ] **C** Is often seen in people with chronic alcohol problems.
- [ ] **D** Is secondary to vitamin B_{12} deficiency.
- [ ] **E** Is irreversible.

3.59 **Duodenal ulcer:**

- [ ] **A** Is associated with normal acid secretion.
- [ ] **B** Can be related to Crohn's disease.
- [ ] **C** Is more prevalent than gastric ulcers.
- [ ] **D** Is usually found in the first part of the duodenum.
- [ ] **E** Is a rare cause of upper gastrointestinal haemorrhage.

3.60 **The following are causes of duodenal ulcers:**

- [ ] **A** *Helicobacter pylori*.
- [ ] **B** Schistosomiasis.
- [ ] **C** Coeliac disease.
- [ ] **D** ACE (angiotensin-converting enzyme) inhibitors.
- [ ] **E** Hyperparathyroidism.

3.57 Answer: C, D, E

TPN supplies all the patient's daily nutritional requirements. A peripheral vein may be used, but longer periods of use with concentrated solutions can readily lead to thrombosis, so central venous access is usually required. General indications for TPN are that patients require long-term (> 10 days) supplemental nutrition because either they are unable to receive all of their daily energy, protein and other nutrient requirements through oral or enteral feeding or they require total nutrition as a result of severe gut dysfunction or inability to tolerate enteral feeding.

Hypo-/hypercalcaemia, hypo-/hyperglycaemia (uncontrolled hyperglycaemia during TPN is probably the most common cause of serious hypernatraemia), hyperchloraemia, trace element and folate deficiency, hypo-/hyperphosphataemia, hypo-/hypermagnesaemia and hypo-/hyperkalaemia, and hypo-/hypernatraemia are recognised complications of TPN. Liver dysfunction evidenced by elevations of transaminases, bilirubin and ALP is common at the start, but these elevations are usually transitory. Non-metabolic complications include pneumothorax, haematoma, thromboembolism and catheter-related sepsis.

3.58 Answer: A, B, C

Wernicke–Korsakoff syndrome is the result of dietary deficiency of thiamine and is reversible. Korsakoff's psychosis is an irreversible amnesic syndrome that develops in untreated cases. Alcohol inhibits uptake of thiamine.

3.59 Answer: B, C, D

Duodenal ulcer is associated with acid hypersecretion and commonly results in gastrointestinal haemorrhage.

3.60 Answer: A, C, E

In addition to NSAIDs (non-steroidal anti-inflammatory drugs) and *H. pylori*, hyperparathyroidism, Crohn's disease and coeliac disease are known to be associated with duodenal ulcers. There is no recognised association with schistosomiasis or ACE inhibitors.

3.61　**Serum urea is:**

☐　**A**　Low in dehydration.

☐　**B**　Low in liver disease.

☐　**C**　Never low in starvation.

☐　**D**　High in renal failure.

☐　**E**　High in gout.

3.62　**Following a polya gastrectomy:**

☐　**A**　Megaloblastic anaemia is common.

☐　**B**　There is an increased risk of gastric malignancy.

☐　**C**　*H. pylori* is eradicated.

☐　**D**　There is an increased risk of pulmonary TB.

☐　**E**　There is folic acid malabsorption.

3.63　**Barrett's oesophagus:**

☐　**A**　Is caused by mutant *p53* over-expression at an early stage in carcinogenesis.

☐　**B**　Is an inherited condition.

☐　**C**　Metaplastic columnar epithelium is pathognomonic.

☐　**D**　Is best treated by Nissen's fundoplication when the condition is associated with hiatus hernia.

☐　**E**　Can be treated with photodynamic therapy.

3.64　**With regard to endocrine gland tumours:**

☐　**A**　Phaeochromocytoma is associated with MEN (multiple endocrine neoplasia) 2.

☐　**B**　Parathyroid gland adenoma is commonly seen in MEN 1.

☐　**C**　Conn's syndrome is caused by adenoma in zona glomerulosa.

☐　**D**　Extra-adrenal phaeochromocytoma produces adrenaline (epinephrine).

☐　**E**　Medullary thyroid carcinoma is associated with MEN 2b.

3.61 Answer: B, D, E

Urea is synthesised in the liver from nitrogen and excreted by the kidneys. In dehydration urea rises in proportion to the creatinine. In renal failure both urea and creatinine rise. Gout may be associated with high urea levels. Urea may rise in early starvation.

3.62 Answer: A, B, D

The megaloblastic anaemia is secondary to loss of intrinsic factor, resulting in vitamin B_{12} deficiency. The increased risk of gastric cancer after a partial gastrectomy is likely to be caused by hypo-/achlorhydria in the remnant. It may also be the result of *H. pylori* in the gastric remnant that is not always eradicated.

3.63 Answer: A, C, E

Barrett's oesophagus is metaplastic columnar epithelium lining the distal epithelium that predisposes to the development of adenocarcinoma. Over-expression of p53 mutant protein is an early event in carcinogenesis. Photodynamic therapy can be used to ablate dysphasia and early cancers. There is no evidence that anti-reflux procedures reverse intestinal metaplasia.

3.64 Answer: A, C, E

MEN 2 includes phaeochromocytoma, medullary carcinoma of thyroid and parathyroid adenoma.

MEN 2b includes multiple mucosal neuromas and a marfanoid appearance.

MEN 1 includes parathyroid gland hyperplasia, pituitary tumour (usually prolactinoma) and pancreatic tumours (usually gastrinomas).

Extra-adrenal phaeochromocytomas do not produce adrenaline because they lack the enzyme PNMT that is present in adrenal gland (they convert noradrenaline [norepinephrine] to adrenaline).

3.65 **In thyroid disorders:**

A Hashimoto's thyroiditis is associated with raised enzyme thyroid peroxidase (TPO).

B Pemberton's sign is a result of retrosternal extension of a multinodular goitre.

C Raised thyroid receptor antibodies are seen in autoimmune thyroiditis.

D Solitary thyroid nodules are often malignant.

E Dysthyroid eye disease can be associated with multinodular goitre.

3.66 **With regard to thyroid malignancy:**

A Medullary carcinoma mostly presents as a nodule that is associated with MEN.

B Most papillary carcinomas are multifocal.

C Follicular carcinoma is slow growing and spreads via blood vessels.

D Thyroid lymphomas are often seen on a background of Hashimoto's thyroiditis.

E Thyroglobulin is a useful tumour marker for all thyroid cancers.

3.67 **With regard to parathyroid glands:**

A Secondary hyperparathyroidism causes hypercalcaemia.

B Primary hyperparathyroidism is always associated with increased calcium excretion.

C Chovstek's sign is carpopedal spasm as a result of hypocalcaemia.

D The most common cause of hypoparathyroidism is postoperative thyroidectomy.

E Acute hypocalcaemia is treated with 10% calcium chloride.

3.68 **With regard to adrenal gland disorders:**

A Hypokalaemia can be a feature of increased cortisol secretion.

B Nelson's syndrome leads to hyperpigmentation of skin and scar tissue.

C Cushing's syndrome is caused by an ACTH-producing tumour of the pituitary gland.

D Conn's syndrome leads to both a raised aldosterone/renin ratio and hyperkalaemia.

E A 1-mg overnight dexamethasone suppression test is the best screening test for Cushing's disease.

3.65 Answer: B, C

Hashimoto's thyroiditis is associated with raised antibodies to TPO. Pemberton's sign is the presence of venous congestion and stridor on elevation of the arm. Solitary thyroid nodules are mostly benign (only 5% are malignant). Dysthyroid eye disease is a feature of Graves' disease and not multinodular goitre.

3.66 Answer: B, C, D

Of medullary carcinomas, 70% are sporadic and present as nodules. Papillary carcinoma spreads through lymph vessels whereas follicular carcinoma spreads via the bloodstream. Thyroglobulin is a useful marker for differentiated thyroid cancer only, i.e. papillary and follicular.

3.67 Answer: B, D, E

Secondary hyperparathyroidism results from hyperphosphataemia and leads to hypocalcaemia. Primary hyperparathyroidism causes increased serum ionised calcium, increased 24-hour calcium excretion and normal ALP. Trousseau's sign is carpopedal spasm induced by placing a tourniquet cuff at 200 mmHg around the upper arm, whereas Chovstek's sign is produced by tapping the facial nerve in front of the auditory meatus to produce a facial contraction. Both are examples of tetany.

3.68 Answer: A, B, E

Nelson's syndrome is grossly elevated ACTH after bilateral adrenalectomy, whereas Cushing's disease is caused by an ACTH-producing tumour in the pituitary gland. Conn's syndrome leads to a raised aldosterone/renin ratio, hypokalaemia and essential hypertension (5%). The 24-h urinary free cortisol is an alternative, less sensitive, screening test for Cushing's disease.

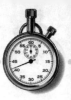

3.69   **With regard to thyroid carcinoma:**

☐ **A** A tumour size < 5 cm in a 30-year-old man has a good prognosis.

☐ **B** Papillary carcinoma has a bad prognosis.

☐ **C** Hoarseness of voice after thyroidectomy is a result of superior laryngeal nerve palsy.

☐ **D** The most common complication of thyroid surgery is recurrent laryngeal nerve palsy.

☐ **E** A 'hot nodule' in a ^{99m}Tc isotope scan may indicate a solitary toxic adenoma.

3.70   **With regard to salivary gland pathology:**

☐ **A** Sialolithiasis is more common in Wharton's duct.

☐ **B** Mumps may affect submandibular as well as sublingual glands.

☐ **C** The most common cause of postoperative parotitis is *Streptococcus* spp.

☐ **D** Sialorrhoea can result from oesophageal obstruction.

☐ **E** Chronic parotitis is caused by dilatation of the duct system.

3.71   **In salivary gland tumours:**

☐ **A** The most common carcinoma is the adenoid cystic type.

☐ **B** Pleomorphic adenomas are more common in men.

☐ **C** Soft cystic mass presentations are more common in Warthin's tumours.

☐ **D** Pleomorphic adenomas consist of mixed epithelial cells.

☐ **E** Papillary projections are common in Warthin's tumour.

3.72   **With regard to skin pathology:**

☐ **A** A punctum is pathognomonic of a congenital dermoid.

☐ **B** Implantation dermoids are from epithelial cells implanted into subcutaneous tissue.

☐ **C** A strawberry naevus usually regresses on its own when the child is aged 5 years.

☐ **D** Keratoacanthomas are a premalignant condition.

☐ **E** Solar keratosis can lead to squamous carcinoma.

3.69   Answer: A, C, E

Tumours < 5 cm in men aged < 40 years and women aged < 45 years have a good prognosis.

Papillary carcinoma has an excellent prognosis. Hoarseness of voice after thyroidectomy can be the result of a recurrent nerve palsy as well as an external branch of a superior laryngeal nerve palsy.

The most common complication of thyroid surgery is hypocalcaemia (5% of thyroidectomies).

3.70   Answer: A, B, D, E

Sialolithiasis comprises cell debris and calcium and magnesium phosphate, and is rare in parotid glands. *Staphylococcus* spp. are the most common cause of postoperative parotitis and are treated with antibiotics and surgical drainage.

3.71   Answer: A, C, D, E

The most common benign tumour is a pleomorphic adenoma, which has equal sex distribution. In fact all salivary gland tumours have an equal sex distribution, except for Warthin's tumour, which is more common in men. Pleomorphic adenomas are surrounded by a fibrous capsule, but there is no extension beyond this.

3.72   Answer: B, C, E

A punctum is pathognomonic of sebaceous cysts (although up to 50% may not have one). Keratoacanthomas are not a premalignant condition but can resemble squamous carcinoma. Excision in the latter is done for cosmetic reasons and to confirm histology.

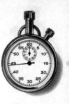

3.73   In skin cancer:

☐   **A**   Malignant melanoma is more common in women.

☐   **B**   Basal cell carcinomas (BCCs) metastasise slowly.

☐   **C**   Squamous cell carcinomas (SCCs) arise from basal cells of the epidermis.

☐   **D**   Superficial spreading melanoma is the most common subtype.

☐   **E**   Breslow's staging measures tumour thickness in millimetres.

3.74   In acute lower limb ischaemia:

☐   **A**   Atrial fibrillation may be a causative factor.

☐   **B**   Thrombus is often seen at the aortic bifurcation.

☐   **C**   Paraesthesia is often the initial symptom.

☐   **D**   Reperfusion injury can lead to compartment syndrome.

☐   **E**   Trauma causes acute ischaemia only in high-risk patients.

3.75   Which of the following are true?

☐   **A**   Buerger's disease is a result of complete thrombotic occlusion of lower limb vessels.

☐   **B**   Mycotic aneurysms are secondary to septic emboli.

☐   **C**   A pseudo-aneurysm is a pulsating haematoma.

☐   **D**   An AAA (aortic artery aneurysm) is saccular in shape.

☐   **E**   Suprarenal AAA repair can cause spinal cord ischaemia.

3.76   The risk factors for arterial thrombosis are:

☐   **A**   Factor V Leiden mutation.

☐   **B**   Hypercholesterolaemia.

☐   **C**   Increased fibrinogen.

☐   **D**   Increased homocysteine.

☐   **E**   Increased platelet count.

3.73   Answer: D, E

Melanoma has equal sex distribution for all adults although for SCCs and BCCs the male/female ratio is 2:1. BCCs never metastasise, preferring local spread. They arise from basal cells of the epidermis whereas SCCs arise from keratinocytes in the epidermis.

3.74   Answer: A, D

Emboli (saddle type) are seen near the aortic bifurcation. Pain is often the presenting feature of acute ischaemia, whereas onset of paraesthesia demands immediate treatment. Reperfusion injury is the result of toxic oxygen radicals. Trauma leads to acute ischaemia by dissection of blood through an intimal tear to the media.

3.75   Answer: B, C, E

Buerger's disease is segmental thrombotic occlusion of small and medium vessels of lower as well as upper limb vessels. AAAs are fusiform in shape. Thoracic and cerebral aneurysms are saccular in shape. Both suprarenal and infrarenal AAA repair can cause spinal cord ischaemia.

3.76   Answer: B, C, D, E

Leiden mutation causes deep venous thrombosis (DVT). Increased homocysteine causes both arterial and venous thrombosis.

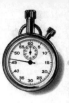

3.77 **In DVT:**

◻ A Phlegmasia alba dolens is the result of thrombosis of lymph vessels.

◻ B Mechanical prophylaxis is preferred over pharmacological prophylaxis in neurosurgery.

◻ C Duration of prophylaxis for postoperative proximal DVT is 6 months.

◻ D Low-molecular-weight (LMW) heparin is better than unfractionated heparin in DVT prophylaxis.

◻ E Heparin-induced thrombocytopenia causes only venous thrombosis.

3.78 **Postphlebitic limb:**

◻ A Typically develops within a month of DVT.

◻ B Gives rise to secondary varicose veins and incompetent perforators.

◻ C Can result in formation of ulcers at the lateral malleolus.

◻ D Has a pathophysiology caused by venous hypertension, which leads to chronic oedema.

◻ E Has antibiotics and limb elevation as the mainstay treatment.

3.79 **In resuscitation:**

◻ A A drop in supine systolic BP is an early indicator for hypovolaemia.

◻ B The presence of palpable carotid indicates systolic BP of at least 60 mmHg.

◻ C A venous cut-down may be performed at the saphenous vein anterior to the medial malleolus.

◻ D Drugs for resuscitation can be given through the intraosseous route.

◻ E Internal cardiac massage can be performed in severe blunt trauma.

3.80 **With regard to acid–base balance:**

◻ A Bicarbonate therapy may induce hyponatraemia and hypo-osmolarity.

◻ B High negative base excess indicates metabolic acidosis.

◻ C Increased CO_2 tension causes a right shift of the oxygen dissociation curve.

◻ D Oxygen saturation indicates the amount of oxygen flowing in the tissues.

◻ E Lactic acid is mainly excreted from the lungs as CO_2.

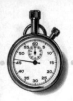

3.77 Answer: B, C, D

Phlegmasia alba dolens is thrombosis of the iliofemoral vessels, often seen in pregnancy.

Graduated elastic compression stockings are an example of mechanical prophylaxis used in neuro- and ophthalmic surgery. Heparin-induced thrombocytopenia is seen with heparin given by any route when 4–15 days into therapy. It causes both arterial and venous thrombosis.

3.78 Answer: B, D

Postphlebitic limb typically develops 1–30 years after thrombosis. It leads to venous ulceration that is typically seen at the medial malleolus. Graduated compression stockings and limb elevation are the mainstays of treatment.

3.79 Answer: B, C, D

Postural hypotension, tachycardia and tachypnoea are early signs of hypovolaemia. Supine hypotension means loss of at least 30% blood volume. The intraosseous route is one of the quickest ways to establish access for the rapid infusion of fluids, drugs and blood products in emergency situations, as well as for resuscitation, and is used in children aged < 7 years. All commonly used drugs for resuscitation can be used except for bicarbonate and bretyllium. Internal cardiac massage is done only for penetrating trauma.

3.80 Answer: B, C, E

Bicarbonate therapy induces hypernatraemia, hyperosmolarity and paradoxical acidosis.

Increases in acidosis, temperature, CO_2 tension and 2,3-DPG (2,3-diphosphoglycerate) all lead to a right shift of the oxygen dissociation curve. The amount of oxygen flowing in the tissues depends on the saturation, cardiac output and haemoglobin. Lactic acid is excreted by the liver and kidney.

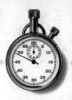

3.81   In trauma:

☐ **A** The tertiary effects of blast injury are caused by the dynamic force of the wind.

☐ **B** CSF rhinorrhoea is commonly associated with Le Fort type I fractures.

☐ **C** The spleen is the most common solid organ injured in blunt injury.

☐ **D** Mesenteric tears are most common at the duodenojejunal flexure.

☐ **E** Bruising in the flank may indicate retroperitoneal haematoma.

3.82   In the metabolic response to trauma:

☐ **A** Necrobiosis can occur directly after the acute ebb phase.

☐ **B** ACTH and cortisol level are both increased in the ebb phase.

☐ **C** During the flow phase, the metabolic rate is comparatively decreased.

☐ **D** In the flow phase, skeletal muscle growth increases.

☐ **E** Insulin resistance is seen in both the ebb and the flow phases.

3.83   In repair of bones and nerves:

☐ **A** Primary callus results from osteo-progenitor cells in the periosteum.

☐ **B** External callus leads to membranous bone formation.

☐ **C** Weight bearing stimulates growth factors and healing.

☐ **D** Wällerian degeneration and chromatolysis are seen in axonotemesis.

☐ **E** Tinel's sign is used to monitor progress in recovery of axon injury.

3.84   In compartment syndrome:

☐ **A** Absent pulse pressure in the distal limb can be an initial feature.

☐ **B** Increased pain during passive flexion and extension rules it out.

☐ **C** Monitoring absolute pressure values are unreliable.

☐ **D** Lower limbs are commonly affected.

☐ **E** Expansion of the compartment as a result of haemorrhage is a causative factor.

3.81 Answer: A, C, D, E

CSF rhinorrhoea is usually associated with Le Fort III fractures. Mesenteric tears are most common at the duodenojejunal flexure and the ileocaecal junction. The presence of bruising in the flank in cases of trauma indicates retroperitoneal haematoma and is also known as Grey Turner's sign.

3.82 Answer: A, B, E

If the ebb phase is not properly managed, necrobiosis sets in directly. During the flow phase the metabolic rate is increased to at least twice normal and skeletal muscle breakdown sets in.

3.83 Answer: A, C, D, E

Primary callus leads to membranous bone formation. External callus is formed from surrounding pluripotent cells. Wällerian degeneration is the distal degeneration of the axon.

3.84 Answer: C, D, E

Pain and paraesthesia are early features, whereas loss of pulses is a very late feature. Increased pain produced by passive flexion and extension indicates a compartment syndrome. Absolute pressures are unreliable. A difference in pressure of < 30 mmHg between diastolic BP and compartment pressure requires immediate fasciotomy.

3.85 **In fat embolism syndrome:**

☐ A The most common cause is penetrating trauma to long bone.

☐ B Caused by high-density lipoproteins (HDLs), very-low-density lipoproteins (VLDLs), LDLs and triglycerides.

☐ C Diagnosed by finding fat globules in retinal vessels and urine.

☐ D The classic triad involves neurological deficit, petechial rash and respiratory failure.

☐ E Sudan black is used to stain fat globules.

3.86 **In burns:**

☐ A Deep partial-thickness burns are often painless.

☐ B Superficial burns may have blisters.

☐ C Hypertrophic scar formation may be seen in partial-thickness burns.

☐ D Full-thickness burns may heal by epithelialisation from pilosebaceous glands.

☐ E Third-space fluid loss is seen in burns.

3.87 **In perioperative assessment:**

☐ A Elective surgery in patients with unstable angina should be delayed.

☐ B Anticoagulation and cardioversion are often successful in atrial flutter.

☐ C Mobitz type 2 block is more severe than type 1 block.

☐ D Adrenaline can be used urgently when a pacemaker has failed.

☐ E Diathermy is contraindicated in patients with a pacemaker.

3.88 **Drugs that do NOT require modification in use before major surgery include:**

☐ A Oral contraceptive pills during abdominal surgery.

☐ B Warfarin.

☐ C Levodopa.

☐ D Insulin.

☐ E Steroids.

3.85 Answer: C, D, E

The most common cause is a blunt trauma leading to a long bone fracture. It is caused by fat globules containing VLDLs and plasma triglycerides.

3.86 Answer: C, E

Partial-thickness burns are painful and blisters are often seen. Superficial burns never form blisters. Full-thickness burns heal by epithelialisation from the wound edges only, whereas partial-thickness burns heal from pilosebaceous glands.

3.87 Answer: A, B, C, D

Diathermy can be used in patients with a pacemaker.

3.88 Answer: none of them

Oral contraceptive pills should be stopped a month before abdominal or pelvic surgery.

Stop warfarin and switch to heparin before surgery.

Omit levodopa before surgery.

It may be necessary to switch to a sliding scale in patients taking insulin. Hydrocortisone is given to patients taking steroids in the perioperative period.

3.89 In anaemia:

A Iron-binding capacity is reduced in anaemia of chronic disease.

B Both MCV (mean cell volume) and MCH (mean cell haemoglobin) are normal in thalassaemia trait.

C The most common cause of anaemia in surgical patients is haemorrhage.

D Hyperthyroidism causes microcytic anaemia.

E Anaemia of chronic disease can be treated with erythropoietin.

3.90 With regard to transfusion reactions:

A Hyperkalaemia and hypercalcaemia are the common electrolyte abnormalities.

B In delayed haemolytic transfusion reaction haemolysis is extravascular.

C Non-haemolytic febrile transfusion reaction is seen after 24 h.

D The lab test for transfusion reaction shows a positive direct anti-globulin test.

E Leukodepletion of all blood products will prevent variant Creutzfeldt–Jakob disease (vCJD).

3.91 With regard to nutritional support:

A Serum transferrin and lymphocyte count are used to assess nutritional state.

B In the postoperative period enteral nutrition maintains gut barrier function.

C Nitrogen balance can be calculated from the urinary nitrogen loss.

D Hyperthyroidism can lead to gastric atony.

E To prevent regurgitation nasogastric tubes should be placed beyond the pylorus.

3.92 With regard to regional anaesthesia:

A Myelinated nerve fibres are blocked earlier than unmyelinated ones.

B 'A' fibres are more sensitive than 'C' fibres to local anaesthesia.

C Bupivacaine can be used for intravenous blockade.

D Methaemoglobinaemia is a side effect of cocaine.

E Prilocaine is the safest agent for intravenous blockade.

3.89   Answer: A, D, E

Both MCV and MCH are lowered in thalassaemia trait. The most common cause of anaemia in surgical patients is iron deficiency anaemia (from chronic blood loss) and anaemia of chronic disease.

3.90   Answer: B, D, E

Hyperkalaemia and hypocalcaemia are common electrolyte abnormalities.

Non-haemolytic febrile reactions are generally seen within hours.

The direct anti-globulin test (DAT) is used to detect whether antibodies (or complement) have bound to RBC surface antigens in vivo. The patient's RBCs are washed and then incubated with anti-human globulin. If immunoglobulin or complement factors have been fixed on to the RBC surface in vivo, the anti-human globulin will agglutinate the RBCs and the direct Coombs' test will be positive.

3.91   Answer: A, B, C, E

Hypothyroidism leads to gastric atony.

3.92   Answer: A, E

'C' fibres are more sensitive than 'A' fibres to local anaesthesia. C fibres carry pain sensation.

Bupivacaine is cardiotoxic and hence not indicated for intravenous blockade.

Prilocaine is the safest for intravenous blockade because of its high therapeutic index. Methaemoglobinaemia, an uncommon disorder (in which haemoglobin is not oxidised and not capable of binding oxygen), is a side effect of prilocaine.

3.93 **Which of the following prevents infection in surgical practice?**

A Laminar airflow in the operating theatre.

B Negative pressure ventilation system in the operating theatre.

C Shaving the operative site with a clean blade 48 h before surgery.

D Use of prophylactic antibiotics for a clean wound in patients with valvular heart disease.

E Sterilisation of the flexible endoscope with 2% glutaraldehyde.

3.94 **With regard to surgical scars:**

A Incisions across Langers' line increase the risk of hypertrophic scars.

B Keloids are more common on the face and deltopectoral region.

C Both hypertrophic scars and keloids can grow beyond the margins of the original wound.

D Simple excision is used to treat hypertrophic scars.

E Increased lysis of collagen is seen only in hypertrophic scars.

3.95 **Which of the following are true with regard to the biology of skin healing?**

A The inflammatory response is mediated by neutrophils and macrophages.

B Angiogenesis stops once the wound is covered with granulation tissue.

C Wound closure is the last step in wound healing.

D Scar contraction is seen in a normal mature scar.

E Fetal skin does not scar as a result of reduced transforming growth factor β_1 (TGF-β_1).

3.96 **With regard to skin grafts:**

A A graft initially derives nourishment from the host by imbibing.

B Granulation tissue is a good recipient for skin graft.

C Split thickness graft consists of epidermis only.

D Full-thickness graft contracts minimally and gives a good colour match.

E Flaps are detached tissue with an artery, veins and capillaries.

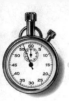

3.93 Answer: A, D, E

Positive pressure ventilation with pressure decreasing from the operating theatre to the anaesthetic room helps to carry micro-organisms out of the room. Shaving of the operative site increases the risk of infection and hence, if necessary, should be performed as near as possible to the time of operation.

3.94 Answer: A, B, E

Only keloids grow beyond the original wound boundary. Hypertrophic scars mostly regress by 6 months and generally require no treatment.

3.95 Answer: A, B, E

Tissue remodelling is the last step of skin healing. Other steps are inflammatory response, granulation tissue formation, angiogenesis and wound closure. Scar contraction is seen when healing has failed in large wounds. Keloids and normal mature wounds do not show scar contraction.

3.96 Answer: A, B, D, E

Split-thickness grafts contain epidermis and a variable amount of dermis.

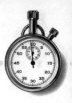

3.97 **With regard to cancer pathogenesis:**

☐   **A**   A proto-oncogene, when activated, gives rise to cancer.

☐   **B**   Apoptosis prevents damaged DNA from passing to the next generation.

☐   **C**   Regulatory control of the cell cycle is lost among cancer cells.

☐   **D**   Inherited gene mutations are the most common cause of cancer.

☐   **E**   Loss of E-cadherin leads to metastasis.

3.98 **With regard to tumour markers:**

☐   **A**   In the early stages of cancer, tumour markers are generally less sensitive.

☐   **B**   CA-19.9 is associated with breast cancer.

☐   **C**   Ca-125 is associated with ovarian cancer.

☐   **D**   Calcitonin is associated with medullary carcinoma of thyroid.

☐   **E**   S-100 is associated with small cell carcinoma of the lung.

3.99 **The acute phase reactants that do NOT increase during the acute phase are:**

☐   **A**   Ceruloplasmin.

☐   **B**   C-reactive protein (CRP).

☐   **C**   Fibrinogen.

☐   **D**   Transferrin.

☐   **E**   Albumin.

3.100 **Which of the following changes occur after surgery?**

☐   **A**   Hypothermia.

☐   **B**   Mild tachycardia.

☐   **C**   Hypoxaemia.

☐   **D**   Adynamic ileus.

☐   **E**   Metabolic alkalosis.

3.97   Answer: B, C, E

A proto-oncogene is a normal gene that has a positive effect on the growth of a cell. Most cancers are generated by factors in the environment, not by inherited gene mutations.

3.98   Answer: A, C, D

CA-19.9 is used for pancreatic cancer whereas S-100 is used for melanoma.

3.99   Answer: D, E

Transferrin and albumin decrease during the acute phase; the rest increase.

3.100   Answer: B, C, D, E

Hyperthermia resulting from increased metabolic rate is common. Mild tachycardia and a threefold increase in cardiac output are common. Hypoxaemia is common as a result of decreased forced vital capacity and functional residual capacity. Adynamic ileus is caused by increased sympathetic tone and is temporary. Metabolic alkalosis results from sodium retention and hydrogen excretion.

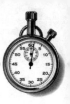

3.101 Biochemical changes that take place after uncomplicated surgery are:

    A Metabolic alkalosis.

    B Hypernatraemia.

    C Right shift of the O_2–haemoglobin dissociation curve.

    D Increased urinary potassium excretion.

    E Increased urinary osmolality.

3.102 Which of the following are true with regard to healing of surgical wounds?

    A The inflammatory response is the key to healing.

    B Haemostasis takes place by the intrinsic pathway only.

    C Granulation tissue is common to all forms of repair.

    D Wound contraction is a feature of healing by secondary intention.

    E Matrix remodelling takes place by 10 days.

3.103 The following nutrients have a role in wound healing:

    A Vitamin A.

    B Zinc.

    C Copper.

    D Vitamin C.

    E Methionine.

3.104 The following are true with regard to tendons and ligaments:

    A Tendons receive their blood supply through vinculae.

    B Ligaments are generally well vascularised.

    C The Achilles' tendon is an example of an avascular tendon.

    D Early passive mobilisation stimulates tendon repair.

    E The anterior cruciate ligament receives its blood supply from the synovial membrane.

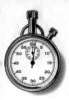

3.101   Answer: A, D, E

After surgery aldosterone, cortisol and vasopressin are secreted, which cause sodium and water retention and metabolic alkalosis. Hyponatraemia occurs as a result of a dilutional effect and an intracellular shift of sodium. Metabolic alkalosis causes a left shift of the dissociation curve.

3.102   Answer: A, C, D, E

Haemostasis takes place by the intrinsic as well as the extrinsic pathways.

3.103   Answer: all true

Vitamins A and C, zinc, copper and protein, especially sulphur-containing amino acids such as methionine, have proven roles in wound healing.

3.104   Answer: A, D, E

Near the attachments of the tendons, folds of connective tissue called vinculae convey blood vessels to the tendons. Ligaments are relatively avascular. Achilles' tendon is an example of a vascular tendon.

3.105 Which of the following describe the mode of action of analgesia?

☐ A NSAIDs prevent the formation of prostaglandins which stimulate nociceptors.

☐ B Opioids block opioid receptors at the dorsal horn of the spinal cord.

☐ C Local anaesthetics block Aδ- and C-fibres.

☐ D Transcutaneous electrical nerve stimulation (TENS) blocks Aβ-fibres.

☐ E Opioids act on the cerebral cortex and change the perception of pain.

3.106 Intravenous opioid patient-controlled analgesia (PCA):

☐ A Is indicated after major surgery in those who are fasting.

☐ B Is contraindicated if there is a history of illicit drug abuse.

☐ C Should not include a loading dose of opioid.

☐ D Is contraindicated in patients with sleep apnoea.

☐ E Can be used where intramuscular injections are contraindicated.

3.107 The following are true with regard to epidural analgesia:

☐ A It reduces incidence of DVT and pulmonary embolism (PE).

☐ B It ran be used for labour pain.

☐ C The side effects include delayed return of gastrointestinal function.

☐ D Respiratory arrest can occur as a complication.

☐ E It reduces postoperative mortality and morbidity.

3.108 With regard to postoperative vomiting:

☐ A Metoclopramide acts on the chemoreceptor trigger zone (CTZ).

☐ B Morphine stimulates the vomiting centre only.

☐ C Pain induces vomiting by stimulating the CTZ.

☐ D Anaesthetic drugs stimulate both the CTZ and the vomiting centre.

☐ E Cyclizine acts on the vomiting centre only.

3.105   Answer: A, C, E

Opioids act as agonists to opioid receptors at the dorsal horn of the spinal cord.

TENS stimulates Aβ-fibres, which inhibit transmission of pain to higher centres.

3.106   Answer: A, B, D, E

A loading dose of opioid must be given. Background infusions are no longer recommended.

3.107   Answer: A, B, D, E

Early return of gastrointestinal function after abdominal surgery is one of the benefits of epidural analgesia.

3.108   Answer: A, D, E

Morphine stimulates both the CTZ and the vomiting centre. Pain induces vomiting by stimulating the vomiting centre.

3.109 Which of the following are true with regard to afterload?

- [ ] A Afterload is decreased by positive intrathoracic pressure.
- [ ] B Rewarming hypothermic patients increases afterload.
- [ ] C Cardiac output is directly proportional to afterload.
- [ ] D Afterload can be defined as systolic ventricular wall tension.
- [ ] E Intra-aortic balloon counterpulsation decreases afterload.

3.110 Which of the following is/are a sign of inadequate tissue perfusion?

- [ ] A Confusion.
- [ ] B Oliguria.
- [ ] C Respiratory rate of 12.
- [ ] D Systolic BP of 100 mmHg.
- [ ] E Capillary refill time of 4 s.

3.111 Which of the following MIGHT indicate respiratory distress?

- [ ] A Tachypnoea.
- [ ] B Confusion.
- [ ] C $Spo_2 < 90\%$.
- [ ] D Inability to complete half a sentence.
- [ ] E Use of sternocleidomastoids during inspiration.

3.112 Blood platelets help to arrest bleeding by:

- [ ] A Releasing factors that promote clotting.
- [ ] B Adhering together to form plugs on exposure to collagen.
- [ ] C Releasing serotonin to cause vasoconstriction.
- [ ] D Releasing high levels of calcium.
- [ ] E Inhibiting the conversion of plasminogen to plasmin.

3.113 Which of the following are used to treat hyperkalaemia?

- [ ] A Calcium resonium orally.
- [ ] B 10% calcium chloride.
- [ ] C Physiological saline (20 ml of 5% solution) and insulin.
- [ ] D 8% sodium bicarbonate.
- [ ] E Intravenous salbutamol.

3.109 Answer: A, D, E

Rewarming hypothermic patients causes vasodilatation, which decreases afterload.

Cardiac output is inversely related to afterload.

3.110 Answer: A, B, E

Tachypnoea and systolic BP < 90 mmHg are signs of tissue hypoperfusion.

3.111 Answer: all true

3.112 Answer: A, B, C

At sites of blood vessel injury, platelets adhere to exposed subendothelial collagen. The main mediator of this adhesion is von Willebrand's factor (vWF), which adheres to platelet membrane GPIb. Initial platelet binding results in upgrading of membrane GPIIb/IIIa receptors that also interact with vWF, allowing stronger binding to collagen and enabling platelets to aggregate. After activation, platelets have two major mechanisms to recruit additional platelets to the growing haemostatic plug. They release pro-aggregatory materials (e.g. ADP) by the release reaction and synthesise thromboxane A_2 from arachidonic acid. This consolidates the initial haemostatic plug by promoting the participation of other platelets. High calcium levels are not needed for haemostasis; normal levels are adequate. Serotonin from platelets can release plasminogen activators.

3.113 Answer: A, B, E

Intravenous dextrose (50 ml of 50% solution) and insulin (6 units) are used. Sodium bicarbonate, if used, is used at the concentration of 1.26%. Both promote a shift of potassium into the intracellular space.

3.114 Which of the following signs indicate ECF volume loss?

- ☐ A Rising haematocrit.
- ☐ B Falling body weight.
- ☐ C Postural hypotension.
- ☐ D Tachycardia.
- ☐ E Fourth heart sound.

3.115 The following steps are correct during cardiac arrest:

- ☐ A Defibrillating three times in pulseless ventricular tachycardia (VT).
- ☐ B Adrenaline is the first drug of choice in asystole.
- ☐ C The dose of adrenaline in ventricular fibrillation (VF) is 2 mg, through the endotracheal tube.
- ☐ D 3 mg intravenous atropine can be given to adults with asystole.
- ☐ E 200 mg lidocaine is used for VF resistant to 3-DC shocks.

3.116 Which of the following causes cardiogenic shock during trauma?

- ☐ A Air embolus.
- ☐ B Cardiac tamponade.
- ☐ C Tension pneumothorax.
- ☐ D Direct myocardial injury.
- ☐ E Trauma-induced myocardial infarction.

3.117 The following parameters can be used to monitor organ perfusion:

- ☐ A Arterial blood gas.
- ☐ B Mixed venous oxygen saturation.
- ☐ C Intestinal mucosal pH.
- ☐ D Temperature.
- ☐ E Urine output.

3.114 Answer: A, B, C, D

Presence of a fourth heart sound may indicate fluid overload.

3.115 Answer: A, B, C, D

The dose of lidocaine in shock-resistant VF is 100 mg.

The new resus council guidelines (2005) state that ventricular fibrillation pulseless VT should be treated with a single shock, followed by immediate resumption of CPR (30 compressions to 2 ventilations). After 2 minutes the rhythm is checked and another shock is given (if indicated).

3.116 Answer: A, B, D, E

Tension pneumothorax is an independent cause of shock.

3.117 Answer: all true

Mixed venous oxygen saturation indicates overall tissue perfusion and organ perfusion. It is measured by pulmonary artery catheterisation.

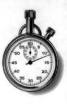

3.118 With regard to transfusion reaction, the following are correct:

- [ ] **A** Mismatch of blood transfusions usually cause anaphylaxis.
- [ ] **B** Rigors are commonly the result of infection.
- [ ] **C** Urticaria is caused by antibodies to plasma protein.
- [ ] **D** Fever can result from anti-leukocyte antibodies.
- [ ] **E** Transfusion-related acute lung injury is caused by sepsis.

3.119 Complications of fractures include:

- [ ] **A** Myositis ossificans.
- [ ] **B** Fat embolism.
- [ ] **C** Sudek's atrophy.
- [ ] **D** Endarteritis obliterans.
- [ ] **E** Volkman's ischaemic contracture.

3.120 With regard to hip pathology, which of the following statements are true?

- [ ] **A** Slipped upper femoral epiphysis is commonly bilateral.
- [ ] **B** Perthes' disease is a self-limiting disorder.
- [ ] **C** In slipped upper femoral epiphysis, the femoral head 'slips' anteriorly.
- [ ] **D** Family history is more common in Perthes' disease.
- [ ] **E** Septic arthritis can cause 'irritable hip'.

3.121 Causes of primary lung damage are:

- [ ] **A** Pneumonia.
- [ ] **B** Aspiration.
- [ ] **C** Smoke inhalation.
- [ ] **D** Pancreatitis.
- [ ] **E** Abdominal sepsis.

3.118   Answer: C, D

Mismatch of blood transfusions from ABO incompatibility causes acute haemolytic transfusion reaction. Anaphylaxis results from reaction to plasma constituents. Transfusion-related acute lung injury is caused by anti-leukocyte antibodies.

3.119   Answer: A, B, C, E

Obliterans arteritis is not associated with fractures.

3.120   Answer: B, E

Slipped femoral epiphysis is bilateral in 20% cases and the family history is positive in 5% of them. The femoral head slips posteriorly in slipped femoral epiphysis.

3.121   Answer: A, B, C

Pancreatitis and abdominal sepsis cause secondary lung damage.

3.122 The following mechanisms lead to hepatocellular jaundice:

    A   Failure of conjugation.

    B   Impaired uptake by hepatocytes.

    C   Excess bilirubin production.

    D   Impaired secretion of conjugated bile in bile canaliculi.

    E   Impairment of bile flow subsequent to secretion by hepatocytes.

3.123 Diagnostic tests used to confirm brain death include:

    A   Fixed pupils not reacting to light.

    B   Absence of corneal reflex.

    C   Absent vestibulo-ocular reflex.

    D   Absent EEG changes even after brain stimulation.

    E   Absent spinal reflexes.

3.124 Which of the following causes raised intracranial pressure (ICP):

    A   Hypoxia.

    B   Hypercapnia.

    C   Hypernatraemia.

    D   Fever.

    E   Sinus thrombosis.

3.125 Which of the following changes may occur in the crush syndrome?

    A   Hyperkalaemia.

    B   Hypercalcaemia.

    C   Raised creatine kinase.

    D   Increased platelet count.

    E   Metabolic acidosis.

3.126 Common nutritional deficiencies are:

    A   Folic acid after gastrectomy.

    B   Vitamin E in pancreatic disease.

    C   Iron in coeliac disease.

    D   Pyridoxine in people who abuse alcohol.

    E   Folate in vegans.

3.122 Answer: A, B, D, E

Excess bilirubin production leads to haemolytic jaundice. Impairment of bile flow, subsequent to secretion by hepatocytes, leads to obstructive jaundice.

3.123 Answer: A, B, C

EEGs are no longer used to diagnose brain death. Spinal reflexes may be present in brain death.

3.124 Answer: A, B, D, E

Hyponatraemia causes increased ICP.

3.125 Answer: A, C, E

Hypocalcaemia and thrombocytopenia occur in the crush syndrome.

3.126 Answer: B, C, D

Vitamin B_{12} deficiency is seen both in vegans and after gastrectomy.

3.127 The following may be a cause of postoperative paralytic ileus:

- A Ganglion blockers.
- B Immobilisation.
- C Peritonitis.
- D Retroperitoneal injury.
- E Uncomplicated laparotomy – commonly seen after.

3128 Which of the following statements are true with respect to tourniquet use?

- A Tourniquets can precipitate sickle cell crises.
- B The reperfusion period can exceed 180 min from the time of application.
- C Previous DVT is a relative contraindication for the lower limb.
- D Cuff pressure should be > 100 mmHg systolic pressure in the upper limb.
- E Tourniquets can be used for finger surgery.

3.129 Pao_2:

- A Decreases in severe anaemia.
- B Decreases at high altitude.
- C May decrease in pulmonary atelectasis.
- D Levels < 8 kPa suggest a need for assisted ventilation.
- E Levels < 10 kPa indicate that respiratory failure is present.

3.130 During wound healing:

- A Inflammation is greater in the presence of catgut than of nylon.
- B With absorbable sutures, the wound strength decreases from the time of suturing.
- C In scurvy the wound is weak as a result of the increased activity of collagenase.
- D Collagen lysis is increased in the presence of infection.
- E During collagen synthesis, lysine and proline are directly incorporated into the collagen molecules.

3.127 Answer: A, B, C, D

Stomach and large bowel atony can be seen within 24–48 hours of uncomplicated laparotomy but true paralytic ileus is not seen after uncomplicated surgery.

3.128 Answer: A, C, E

Reperfusion time is about 90 min for the upper limb and 120 min for the lower limb. Cuff pressure should not exceed 75 mmHg and 100 mmHg systolic pressure for the upper and lower limbs, respectively. Special ring tourniquets are available for finger surgery.

3.129 Answer: B, C, D

Arterial oxygen tension is independent of the Hb level. However, tissue delivery of oxygen is compromised in patients with anaemia. Respiratory failure is said to be present when $Pao_2 < 8$ kPa.

3.130 Answer: A, B, D

Collagen synthesis is reduced in scurvy because vitamin C (ascorbic acid) is needed for the enzyme protocollagen hydroxylase. During collagen synthesis, lysine and proline are incorporated into the protocollagen molecules, which are then acted on by protocollagen hydroxylase.

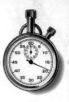

3.131 **In ionising radiation:**

- [ ] **A** Cells in the G1 phase of the cell cycle are most sensitive.
- [ ] **B** Mitosis occurs in irradiated cells.
- [ ] **C** Cells experiencing hypoxia are vulnerable to radiation damage.
- [ ] **D** Granulation tissue formation is delayed in wounds that have been radiated.
- [ ] **E** Undifferentiated tumours are usually more sensitive to radiation than differentiated ones.

3.132 **The following definitions are correct:**

- [ ] **A** Hypoplasia – abnormal growth of an organ.
- [ ] **B** Aplasia – failure of differentiation of an embryonic cell mass into organ-specific tissue.
- [ ] **C** Metaplasia – transformation of one type of mature differentiated cell type into another type.
- [ ] **D** Agenesis – failure of formation of an embryonic mass.
- [ ] **E** Atrophy – decrease in the size of an organ as a consequence of reduction in cell size.

3.133 **Compared with benign tumours, neoplastic tumours show:**

- [ ] **A** Nuclear hyperchromatism.
- [ ] **B** Uniform cell mass.
- [ ] **C** Disproportionately large nuclei relative to cell cytoplasm.
- [ ] **D** Variable shape and size.
- [ ] **E** High mitotic index.

3.134 **Granulomatous inflammation:**

- [ ] **A** Is a type IV hypersensitivity response.
- [ ] **B** Shows dominant infiltration of tissue by plasma cells.
- [ ] **C** Contains epithelioid cells derived from tissue histiocytes.
- [ ] **D** Occurs in sarcoidosis.
- [ ] **E** Is a feature of mycobacterial infection.

3.131 Answer: B, D, E

Cells are most vulnerable in mitosis whereas they are most resistant in G1.

Mitosis still occurs with radiation. Hypoxia appears to protect against radiation. The centre of a malignant tumour is protected by hypoxia.

3.132 Answer: B, C, D, E

Hypoplasia refers to the incomplete growth of an organ or part resulting in a failure of the organ to mature or reach normal size.

3.133 Answer: A, C, D, E

Uniform cell mass is a feature of benign tumours.

3.134 Answer: A, C, D, E

T cells and macrophages predominantly infiltrate areas of granulomatous inflammation.

3.135 Following an injury to a peripheral nerve:

☐ **A** There is degeneration of axon and myelin proximal to the damage.

☐ **B** There is proliferation of Schwann cells in the distal cells.

☐ **C** There is often loss of sweating in the area of skin supplied by the nerve.

☐ **D** Central chromatolysis is a feature.

☐ **E** Sprouting of axons occurs in the stump of the proximal axon.

3.136 Causes of a slow pulse (< 50 bpm) include:

☐ **A** Raised ICP.

☐ **B** Anaemia.

☐ **C** Hypothermia.

☐ **D** Vasovagal episodes.

☐ **E** May be normal in very fit people.

3.135   Answer: B, C, D, E

The classification of nerve injury described by Seddon comprised neurapraxia, axonotmesis and neurotmesis.

A first-degree injury or neurapraxia involves a temporary conduction block with demyelination of the nerve at the site of injury. Once the nerve has remyelinated at that area, complete recovery occurs. Recovery may take up to 12 weeks.

A second-degree injury or axonotmesis results from a more severe trauma or compression. This results in Wällerian degeneration distal to the level of injury and proximal axonal degeneration to at least the next node of Ranvier. Axonal regeneration occurs at the rate of 1 mm/day and can be monitored with an advancing Tinel's sign. The endoneurial tubes remain intact and, therefore, recovery is complete with axons.

Third-degree injury or neurotmesis is the separation of the axon and is the most advanced involvement. Regeneration occurs at 1 mm/day, and progress may be monitored with an advancing Tinel's sign. However, with the increased severity of the injury, the endoneurial tubes are not intact, and regenerating axons may therefore not reinnervate the original motor and sensory targets.

Loss of sweating, coolness, some degree of cyanosis and swelling result from the autonomic disturbance that accompanies many major complete peripheral nerve injuries.

3.136   Answer: A, C, D, E

Physiological causes of increased vagal tone include the bradycardia seen in athletes. Pathological causes include inferior wall myocardial infarction, toxic or environmental exposure, electrolyte disorders, infection, sleep apnoea, drug effects, hypoglycaemia, hypothyroidism and increased ICP. A slow pulse may be caused by many stimuli including cervical dilatation and traction on the eyeball. Unopposed neostigmine causes bradycardia. Anaemia is usually accompanied by a tachycardia.

Single best answer questions

3.137 After an aspirin overdose, which of the following statements is false?

    ☐ **A** Potassium excretion is increased.

    ☐ **B** Respiratory alkalosis is an early finding.

    ☐ **C** Metabolic acidosis is not seen in children.

    ☐ **D** Insensible fluid losses are increased.

    ☐ **E** Tinnitus is a complication.

3.138 With regard to oesophageal cancer:

    ☐ **A** Gastro-oesophageal reflux disease (GORD) usually leads to Barrett's oesophagus.

    ☐ **B** Barrett's oesophagus is usually an incidental finding.

    ☐ **C** Barrett's oesophagus increases the risk of squamous carcinoma.

    ☐ **D** Adenocarcinomas of the oesophagus are radiosensitive.

    ☐ **E** Tracheo-oesophageal fistula is the most common cause of respiratory symptoms.

3.139 Which of the following is NOT a risk factor for DVT?

    ☐ **A** Obesity.

    ☐ **B** Oral contraceptive pill.

    ☐ **C** Immobility.

    ☐ **D** Nephrotic syndrome.

    ☐ **E** Dipyridamole.

3.140 With regard to renal cell carcinoma, which of the following statements is false?

    ☐ **A** Stage II tumours are contained within Gerota's fascia.

    ☐ **B** The tumours may cause polycythaemia.

    ☐ **C** They commonly present with flank pain.

    ☐ **D** Liver metastases are more common than lung metastases.

    ☐ **E** Renal transplantation is a risk factor.

3.137 Answer: C

Aspirin overdose gives rise to an initial respiratory alkalosis followed by a metabolic acidosis. The alkalosis may be transient in children and metabolic acidosis may therefore occur at an earlier stage. The excretion of potassium, bicarbonate and water is increased. Dehydration occurs secondary to vomiting and insensible losses (hyperthermia, tachypnoea).

3.138 Answer: B

GORD leads to the development of Barrett's oesophagus in about 10% of cases. It is usually found incidentally at endoscopy and causes a 30-fold increase in the risk of adenocarcinoma. Adenocarcinomas are not radiosensitive and surgical treatment is required. Respiratory symptoms are most often the result of overspill and only rarely of a fistula.

3.139 Answer: E

Dypiridamole is an anti-platelet agent that is not associated with DVT.

3.140 Answer: D

Renal cell carcinoma metastasises more often to lung and soft tissue than to the liver.

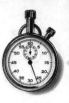

3.141 In calcific tendonitis of the shoulder, which of the following statements is true?

☐ A The biceps tendon is usually calcified.

☐ B The point of maximal tenderness is over the spine of the scapula.

☐ C The pain is of sudden onset.

☐ D External rotation is the main movement to be restricted.

☐ E Passive movements are not restricted.

3.142 The following are ALL true with regard to muscle injury EXCEPT:

☐ A Excessive scar tissue formation may affect movement.

☐ B Active mobilisation favours rapid and complete regeneration.

☐ C Immobilisation increases muscle sensitivity to insulin.

☐ D Ischaemia of muscle can lead to contractures.

☐ E Disuse atrophy occurs in skeletal muscle.

3.143 Which of the following statements is false with regard to thyroid tumours?

☐ A Papillary carcinoma is the most common.

☐ B Medullary carcinoma may be monitored by measuring calcitonin.

☐ C Medullary carcinoma is associated with multiple endocrine neoplasia (MEN) 2.

☐ D Anaplastic carcinoma usually has a poor prognosis.

☐ E Follicular carcinoma is more common in men.

3.144 Gynaecomastia may be seen in all of the following EXCEPT:

☐ A Newborn infants.

☐ B Klinefelter syndrome.

☐ C Hypopituitarism.

☐ D Phenytoin use.

☐ E Turner syndrome.

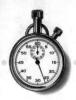

3.141   Answer: C

Calcific tendonitis of the shoulder involves calcification of the supraspinatus tendon. Tenderness is mostly anteromedial and the pain is of sudden onset.

External rotation is preserved but other movements, both passive and active, are restricted.

3.142   Answer: C

Immobilisation decreases muscle sensitivity to insulin and hence less glucose and more lactate accumulate in muscle.

3.143   Answer: E

Follicular carcinomas, as with all thyroid tumours, are more common in women.

3.144   Answer: E

Turner syndrome is a rare chromosomal disorder of females (XO), characterised by short stature, webbed neck and lack of sexual development at puberty.

3.145 Which of the following statements is false with regard to the peripheral blood film?

☐ **A** Basophilic stippling may be seen in lead poisoning.

☐ **B** Spherocytosis is seen in haemolysis.

☐ **C** Burr cells are seen after splenectomy.

☐ **D** Rouleaux formation indicates a high erythrocyte sedimentation rate (ESR).

☐ **E** Macrocytosis occurs in hypothyroidism.

3.146 Which of the following viruses is NOT associated with cancer in humans?

☐ **A** HIV (human immunodeficiency virus).

☐ **B** Hepatitis B virus (HBV).

☐ **C** Human papillomavirus (HPV).

☐ **D** Herpes zoster virus (HZV).

☐ **E** Epstein–Barr virus (EBV).

3.147 Which of the following statements is true with regard to nosocomial infection:

☐ **A** Percutaneous transmission of hepatitis C virus (HCV) is higher than that of HIV and hepatitis B virus (HBV).

☐ **B** HIV can be transmitted through contaminated synovial fluid.

☐ **C** Presence of high antibody level against HBeAg indicates high infectivity.

☐ **D** Post-exposure prophylaxis against HIV should be continued for 6 months.

☐ **E** The carrier rate after adult infection is almost same for HCV and HBV.

3.148 Which of the following is NOT a marker of poor prognosis in Hodgkin's lymphoma?

☐ **A** Pruritis.

☐ **B** Weight loss > 10% in the last 6 months.

☐ **C** Reed–Sternberg cells in the bone marrow.

☐ **D** Lymphocyte-depleted disease.

☐ **E** Night sweats.

3.145 Answer: C

Burr cells are irregularly shaped cells seen in uraemia.

3.146 Answer: D

HIV: Kaposi's sarcoma.
HBV: hepatocellular carcinoma.
HPV: cervical cancer.
HZV: shingles.
EBV: Burkitt's lymphoma and nasopharyngeal carcinoma.

3.147 Answer: B

The transmission rate of HBV is 30%, HCV 10% and HIV < 1%. The presence of HBeAg indicates high infectivity. Post-exposure prophylaxis against HIV is for 1 month and consists of three drugs: zidovudine, lamivudine and nelfinavir. The carrier rate after adult infection with HCV is 80% whereas for HBV it is 5%.

3.148 Answer: A

Symptoms (night sweats, unexplained pyrexia > 38°C or weight loss > 10% in the last 6 months) indicate more extensive disease. Lymphocyte-depleted forms have the worst prognosis.

3.149 With respect to transfusion reactions, which of the following is false?

- ☐ A Anaphylactic reactions are more common in IgA deficiency.
- ☐ B ABO incompatibility causes haemolysis within the spleen.
- ☐ C Clerical error is the most common cause of haemolytic transfusion reaction.
- ☐ D In fluid overload, the transfusion should be slowed or stopped.
- ☐ E Febrile non-haemolytic reactions usually resolve without specific treatment.

3.150 With regard to mechanisms of skin loss, which statement is false?

- ☐ A Contusions result from penetrating trauma.
- ☐ B Infected abrasions, if not cleaned, lead to permanent skin tattooing.
- ☐ C Degloving injury is the result of a severe shearing force on the skin.
- ☐ D Avulsion is complete tearing away of tissue.
- ☐ E Retraction of edges in small lacerations is common in children.

3.151 With regard to lasers, which statement is false?

- ☐ A Laser radiation penetrates deeply into the body.
- ☐ B Collimation allows the beam to be focused into a small spot.
- ☐ C The penetration of the beam into tissue is related to its wavelength.
- ☐ D Coherence means that the waves in the beam are all in step.
- ☐ E Monochromaticity means that all the light is the same wavelength.

3.152 Which is a live vaccine?

- ☐ A Measles.
- ☐ B Yellow fever.
- ☐ C Polio.
- ☐ D Diphtheria.
- ☐ E Rubella.

3.149   Answer: B

ABO incompatibility causes intravascular haemolysis.

3.150   Answer: A

Contusion is seen in blunt trauma. Retraction of the edges in small lacerations is common in children as a result of greater skin elasticity and this makes the wound look larger.

3.151   Answer: A

The word laser is an acronym for light amplification by the stimulated emission of radiation. The 'light' produced by a laser may be in the visible, UV or IR regions of the electromagnetic spectrum. It is distinguished from that coming from other sources by virtue of its spatial coherence (all the waves of light are in step and in phase), monochromaticity (the radiation has a very narrow bandwidth – all of 'one colour') and high collimation (a narrow beam that does not 'spread out' with distance from the source). Laser radiation does not penetrate deeply into the body so it is only the eyes and the skin that need to be protected.

3.152   Answer: D

Live vaccines consist of strains with little pathogenicity. Diphtheria and tetanus are toxoids, i.e. inactivated toxins that do not cause symptoms but are immunogenic. Live vaccines can cause disease in immunocompromised patients.

3.153 Which of the statements is true regarding sterilisation?

☐ **A** Partly inactivates infectious organisms.

☐ **B** May be achieved by autoclaves or irradiation.

☐ **C** Is often achieved using hypochlorite compounds.

☐ **D** Is the method used to prepare the skin before surgery.

☐ **E** Cannot be used for delicate instruments.

3.154 Which statement is true with regard to glycogen synthesis in the liver?

☐ **A** It is activated by adrenaline (epinephrine).

☐ **B** It takes place in the cell cytosol.

☐ **C** It is regulated primarily by substrate control.

☐ **D** It does not occur in the glycogen storage diseases.

☐ **E** It is activated by glucagon.

3.155 Which statement is true about iron absorption?

☐ **A** It is enhanced by acid suppression.

☐ **B** It occurs mostly in the distal ileum.

☐ **C** It occurs mainly in the duodenum and jejunum.

☐ **D** It is inhibited by vitamin C.

☐ **E** It is hardly ever impaired postgastrectomy.

3.156 All of the following coagulation factors are made in the liver, EXCEPT for:

☐ **A** Factor XII.

☐ **B** Factor V.

☐ **C** Von Willebrand's factor.

☐ **D** Prothrombin.

☐ **E** Platelet cofactor I.

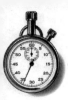

3.153 Answer: B

Sterilisation inactivates all infectious organisms and is usually achieved by autoclaving or irradiation. Delicate instruments can be sterilised using low-pressure steam. Glutaraldehyde can also be used to sterilise instruments if they are adequately cleaned first, provided that the instruments are immersed for a sufficient length of time. Disinfectants are used to prepare the skin before surgery. Hypochlorite compounds are often used to disinfect surfaces/spillage.

3.154 Answer: B

Glucagon and adrenaline both inhibit glycogen synthesis. Glycogen synthesis is regulated by hormonal control primarily. Glycogen storage diseases result in an abnormal type or amount of glycogen.

3.155 Answer: C

Iron is mainly absorbed in the duodenum and upper small intestine. Absorption is impaired in patients with achlorhydria, after partial gastrectomy or in patients on acid-suppressing drugs. Vitamin C keeps iron in a soluble form.

3.156 Answer: C

Factor VIII is synthesised by endothelial cells. As well as being the natural carrier protein for factor VIII, vWF (required for platelet adhesive function) is synthesised in endothelial cells and megakaryocytes.

3.157 A 56-year-old woman presents with fluctuating dysphasia and weight loss over 1 year. She has retrosternal discomfort on eating and weight loss of half a stone. Clinical examination of the neck is normal. The investigation of choice is:

- A Oesophageal manometry.
- B CT of the chest.
- C Barium swallow.
- D Endoscopy.
- E None of the above.

3.158 In trauma:

- A Neurogenic shock causes tachycardia, vasodilatation and hypothermia.
- B Bilateral pulmonary infiltrates are suggestive of acute respiratory distress syndrome (ARDS).
- C The respiratory rate in Cushing's reflex is unaltered.
- D Cerebral perfusion pressure is independent of mean arterial pressure.
- E Good resuscitation may prevent primary brain damage.

3.159 After a road traffic accident:

- A Respiratory failure in someone who is paraplegic can be the result of phrenic nerve palsy.
- B A spiral fracture can be caused by a direct blow.
- C Central spinal cord injury affects the upper limb more than the lower limb.
- D Spinal shock causes spastic paralysis.
- E 'Sacral sparing' is loss of pinprick sensation in the sacral area.

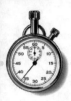

3.157   Answer: D

Manometry may give useful information but an endoscopy is mandatory in dysphasia and weight loss. CT will stage oesophageal cancer but is diagnostically less useful.

3.158   Answer: B

Neurogenic shock involves bradycardia, vasodilatation and loss of temperature control. The respiratory rate in the Cushing's reflex is decreased.

CPP = MAP – ICP

where CPP is cerebral perfusion pressure, MAP is mean arterial pressure and ICP is intracerebral pressure.

Good resuscitation can prevent secondary brain damage. Primary brain damage can be prevented by prevention of the initial trauma.

3.159   Answer: C

Respiratory failure in someone with paraplegia is caused by intercostal muscle failure because the lesion is above T12. In someone with tetraplegia phrenic nerve palsy is seen because the lesion is above C5. Spiral fractures are the result of twisting injury whereas a direct blow causes a transverse fracture.

Spinal shock causes flaccid paralysis, autonomic dysfunction and gastric dilatation.

Sacral sparing involves sparing of the perianal sensation, rectal motor function and great toe flexor activity.

INDEX